UNDERSTANDING OBSESSIONS AND
COMPULSIONS
A self-help manual

Dr Frank Tallis is a writer and practising clinical psychologist. He has held lecturing posts in clinical psychology and neuroscience at the Institute of Psychiatry and King's College London. He is one of the country's leading authorities on obsessional states and played a key role in setting up Obsessive Action (now OCD Action) – a charity for people suffering from obsessive–compulsive disorder and their families. He has written several self-help books (also published by Sheldon), a textbook on obsessive–compulsive disorder, and two psychology books for the general reader: *Changing Minds: A History of Psychotherapy as an Answer to Human Suffering* and *Hidden Minds: A History of Psychotherapy as an Answer to Human Suffering* and *Hidden Minds: A History of the Unconscious*. In 1999 he received a Writers' Award from the Arts Council of Great Britain and in 2000 he won the New London Writers' Award (London Arts Board).

Overcoming Common Problems Series

Selected titles

A full list of titles is available from Sheldon Press,
36 Causton Street, London SW1P 4ST and on our website at
www.sheldonpress.co.uk

Overcoming Common Problems

UNDERSTANDING OBSESSIONS AND COMPULSIONS
A self-help manual

Dr Frank Tallis

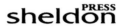

First published in Great Britain in 1992

Sheldon Press
36 Causton Street
London SW1P 4ST

British Library Cataloguing-in-Publication Data
A catalogue record for this book is available from the British Library

ISBN 978–0–85969–652–4

Photoset by Deltatype Ltd, Birkenhead, Wirral
First printed and bound in Great Britain by
Biddles Ltd, King's Lynn, Norfolk
Subsequently digitally
printed in Great Britain

Produced on paper from sustainable forests

Contents

Acknowledgements

I would like to thank Professor Graham Davey for his comments on chapters dealing with learning theory, Ruth Williams for her advice on personality disorder and depression, Dr Ian Jakes and Dr Paul Salkovskis for their consideration of several of the chapters on the treatment of obsessive–compulsive disorder, and Dr E. Higgins for her advice on skin care. I would also like to thank Professor Isaac Marks for his support and helpful criticism while I have been attempting to develop doubt-reduction procedures. A special thank you also to Nicola Fox for reading the completed manuscript and suggesting changes where necessary. I would also like to thank my patients, without whom I could not have written this book. Any deficiencies in the text are of course entirely attributable to the author.

Introduction

The term 'obsession' is a common one. In everyday conversation one is not surprised to hear the word; for example: 'He can't stop thinking about her, he's obsessed!' Further evidence of the term's currency can be found at the perfume counter: look at the labels closely, and 'Obsession' may be one of them! We use the word obsession to mean something that appears to take us over. Something that occupies our minds completely, to the point where everything else seems unimportant. The *Concise Oxford Dictionary* defines an obsession as an 'unreasonably persistent idea in the mind'; however, it is derived from the Latin *obsidere*, meaning 'to besiege'. It is this meaning of the word that can help us to determine whether our thoughts are a serious problem or not. Most people have persistent ideas; however, if those ideas – or our response to those ideas – results in unhappiness and restricted freedom, then some type of treatment might be necessary.

This book is about the self-treatment of obsessional thoughts and compulsive behaviours. But before attempting to undertake treatment, it is necessary to look at the problem in some detail.

In the first chapters I try to answer some basic questions about obsessive–compulsive disorder and obsessive – compulsive personality disorder. For example, what do healthcare specialists like clinical psychologists and psychiatrists mean when they refer to these problems, and how are these problems treated? To answer these questions it will be necessary to learn a little about anxiety and anxiety disorders; it will also be necessary to learn about a particular type of treatment called 'behaviour therapy', and a new version of this called 'cognitive behaviour therapy'.

After reading the first part of this book, you should be able to decide whether or not you have an obsessional problem. If you think you do, then a number of self-help techniques are described in later chapters. Work through the chapters.

A technique called 'exposure and response-prevention' will form the core component of your self-help plan. It is also the most thoroughly tested non-drug treatment for obsessive–compulsive disorder. It will be essential that you understand and practice this particular technique to make progress. Various charts and tables are supplied in the Appendix for you to photocopy for your own personal use.

Overall, several self-help techniques will be described. Not all of them will be applicable, or relevant, to your problem. You may also find that some techniques are more helpful than others. When undertaking a self-help programme, adopt an experimental attitude. If something works for you, then keep it as part of your programme. If, after giving a particular technique a fair chance, you find it doesn't help, then exclude it from your programme. Everyone is different, and different individuals respond to different therapeutic techniques. Nothing in this book should be treated as gospel! You may find that you want to modify some of the techniques. If your modifications improve the treatment's effectiveness, that's fine. Creativity is not only permitted, it is desirable!

If you have more than one obsessional complaint, then don't get overwhelmed. You need only deal with one complaint at a time. Without the support of a therapist, you must be very careful not to take on too much. As a general rule, you can improve your chances of success by setting modest and realistic goals at first. Increase task demands slowly.

Lastly, you are invited to comment on the treatment strategies outlined in the book and to take part in a programme of ongoing research into obsessive–compulsive disorders. (See Appendix V.)

A Treatment Guide for different forms of obsessive–compulsive disorder

All of these treatments are described in this book.

Problem	Treatment
Washing and cleaning	Exposure, self-imposed delay, and response-prevention
	Exposure and response-prevention
Checking	Exposure, self-imposed delay, and response-prevention
	Exposure and response-prevention
	Imaginal exposure
	Doubt reduction procedures 1. distinctive figures and fading 2. distinctive imagery

Primary obsessional slowness	Pacing and prompting
Need for symmetry	Exposure, self-imposed delay, and response-prevention
	Exposure and response-prevention
Hoarding	Exposure, self-imposed delay, and response-prevention
	Exposure and response-prevention
Obsessions and ruminations	Habituation training 1. mental rehearsal 2. written rehearsal 3. use of loop tape
	Thought-stopping Thought-switching Thought-control
Morbid preoccupations and worry	Problem solving Decatastrophizing 1. reason generation 2. being realistic Relaxation Postponement to scheduled worry-time

1

Obsessions

Everyday obsessions

Most people, at some point in their lives, can lay claim to an obsession, or at least to having become 'fixated' on something. The line between serious obsessions, and certain enthusiasms, can be blurred. Take collecting, for example. To anyone who doesn't have an interest in stamps, philately can seem a curiously sterile pursuit. Why would anybody want to spend so much time – and money – collecting small pieces of paper? Can it really be worth it? Occasionally, the keen philatelist might be unable to stop him- or herself from buying a particularly attractive exhibit. Further, such expenditure may even cause domestic conflict because an unsympathetic spouse does not share the collector's interest.

Yet, broadly speaking, most people – even if they don't have an interest in stamps – can see how stamp-collecting might be justified. An attractive stamp could be compared to a small work of art, while a rare stamp might accrue in value. But what about less common 'collectables'? How can the collection of fluffy animals, or tea-towels be justified? Not long ago, a woman was interviewed on a prime-time TV chat-show who collected biscuits! Could people with such unusual interests be considered obsessional in any way?

Another common occurrence with 'obsessional' features is falling in love. When someone falls in love, all s/he wants to do is to think about, talk about, or be with, the person s/he has fallen in love with. The comparison between serious or 'clinical' obsessionality (i.e. obsessionality recognized as a (medical) problem – because it interferes with everyday living) and falling in love is strengthened, by our frequent use of terms such as 'love-sick'. A young man in the throws of love-sickness may lose his appetite, his ability to concentrate, and generally act as though he has been afflicted by some strange illness. In Shakespeare's *Romeo and Juliet*, as soon as Romeo appears, he describes himself as a 'sick man', and makes reference to a 'madness most discreet'.

A more sinister variant of this kind of attachment is jealousy. Suspicion and possessiveness can easily get out of hand, causing continual arguments within an otherwise successful relationship.

Again, Shakespeare (in *Othello*) described this kind of problem long before psychologists, and gave us a new figure of speech to boot: 'O! beware, . . . of jealousy; It is the green-ey'd monster which doth mock The meat it feeds on'. Are people who fall in love, or people who become plagued with suspicion, obsessional – albeit temporarily?

A final example of everyday behaviour that resembles serious obsessionality is excessive devotion to work. An ambitious individual might pursue success with relentless ambition. Being a 'workaholic' might secure a large income or special status, but at the same time leave little time for anything else.

Clearly, then, any kind of extreme and fixed interest could be termed obsessional. Collecting things; developing a crush; becoming jealous; extreme ambition; all have obsessional qualities; they can also interfere with everyday life, to the point where professional help might be needed. However, on the whole, these are all examples of normal behaviour.

When mental healthcare specialists such as psychologists and psychiatrists talk about obsessionality, they have something quite specific in mind. They are usually referring to one of two conditions, either obsessive–compulsive personality disorder, or obsessive–compulsive disorder. These will be briefly described in turn.

Obsessionality as a problem

Personality disorder

'Obsessive–compulsive personality disorder', is the name given to a group of personality characteristics (or traits), which tend to occur together in certain individuals. Strictly speaking, the individual is asymptomatic. That is, there are no particular psychiatric symptoms; such as unusual or repetitive behaviour. Rather, the obsessional personality comprises a pattern of pervasive characteristics.

Characteristics

Perfectionism Perfectionism is normally regarded as a good thing; we very rarely use the term 'perfectionist' in a derogatory way; perfectionists, after all, tend to do things very carefully, and to a very high standard. However, obsessional perfectionism is associated with standards that are set so high, that they actually interfere with the task in hand so that it is not completed. For example, an individual with obsessional perfectionism may be unable to complete decorating his home because he never feels that his work is good enough.

Preoccupation with detail Preoccupation with detail is another obsessional characteristic. The individual may be so concerned with the incidental aspects of a job, that the whole point of it is somehow lost or forgotten. For example, a lecturer may be so concerned that his reading list is not up to date, that he feels unable to give his students their lecture. Another example would be a housewife who decides to start spring cleaning, but ends up spending the whole day scrubbing the inside of her cooker. Preoccupation with rules, lists, order, and organization are also closely associated with excessive concern with detail.

Indecisiveness Here, decision-making is either postponed unnecessarily, or avoided altogether. This difficulty need not be related to important decisions: an obsessional individual may find it difficult to decide what to do when presented with the most trivial of choices – e.g. what sock to put on first.

To these can be added a number of other personality traits or characteristics:

An insistence on doing things in a particular way This insistence is unreasonable and includes a reluctance to let other people attempt tasks just in case they are undertaken incorrectly.

Inability to discard certain possessions even though they are worn out or have no sentimental value.

Overconscientiousness This is often made conspicuous by an inflexible set of morals or values.

Excessive devotion to work This will result in sacrificing leisure time, and being unable to see friends and family.

Difficulty expressing emotions and feelings.

Lack of generosity There is a general resistance to the idea of giving.

Diagnosis

It is not necessary to have all of the above features for a diagnosis of 'obsessive–compulsive personality disorder' to be made. The presence of only five of them, is usually taken to be sufficient to warrant the diagnosis. You can probably think of several people, quite easily, who have five or more of the above characteristics. This might prompt you to ask 'Do they then, need professional help?' The answer is, of course, probably not. A diagnosis is only made when these characteristics interfere with day-to-day living. Furthermore, in most cases where obsessive–compulsive personality disorder can be diagnosed, it is usually not the personality disorder itself which leads to professional involvement, but rather an associated complaint, such as depression.

There are many who question the whole notion of personality disorder. We are all different, and designating clinical diagnoses to individuals who are extreme on certain dimensions of personality might be viewed as nothing more than prejudice. Just because the majority of people conform to something we call a 'normal personality', doesn't necessarily mean that people who don't conform should be given a psychiatric diagnosis. A useful distinction might be made here between 'disturbed' behaviour and 'disturbing' behaviour. It may be that the problem lies in society's intolerance of differences, rather than in the individual him- or herself. In effect, the individual is not disturbed, but rather, society finds him, or her, disturbing.

However, in spite of the above consideration, the evidence tends to suggest that, on the whole, obsessional personality characteristics coincide more often than would be expected by chance alone. But whether we take such evidence as justification for a psychiatric diagnosis is a matter of opinion.

Treatment

The treatment of obsessive–compulsive personality disorder can take many forms. Traditional psychoanalytic therapies have been favoured in the past. However, more recently, an approach called 'cognitive therapy' has been modified so that it can be applied to the treatment of personality problems. It is a 'talking cure' in which the individual learns to alter the way he or she thinks.

Some therapists are now combining aspects of traditional psychoanalysis (where the relationship between the therapist and patient is seen as being central to the process of therapeutic change) with components of cognitive therapy. A good example of this new eclecticism is an approach called 'Schema-focused cognitive therapy'. Here, an attempt is made to change how the patient thinks by challenging unhelpful beliefs, while at the same time recognizing that early events and relationships may have had an important effect on the development of those beliefs. It is, without doubt, far too early to comment on the efficacy of schema-focused cognitive therapy or traditional cognitive therapy as a 'treatment' for obsessive–compulsive personality disorder. Nevertheless, among the numerous psychotherapies currently advocated for personality problems, those that fall beneath the cognitive therapy banner show considerable promise.

Seeking help

If you feel that you might have an obsessional personality problem, and that this is interfering with your life, then you might consider seeking professional help. Your GP could refer you to a clinical psychologist who specializes in cognitive therapy, and he or she may be able to help. However, do remember that the availability of appropriate therapists depends largely on the quality of local resources. Unfortunately, the provision of psychological care is unevenly distributed in Britain, and you may have to spend some time on a waiting list before being seen. You might also need to branch out of your local area. A realistic estimate of therapy duration might be anywhere between six months and two years.

Self-help

Some of the characteristics of obsessive–compulsive personality disorder are also associated with obsessive–compulsive disorder. Suggestions which might help to modify a few of these characteristics are given later in this book (see Chapter 10). However, it should be noted that these are simply suggestions, and nothing more. They are not a satisfactory treatment for obsessive-compulsive personality disorder, which is best dealt with in therapy.

Obsessive–compulsive disorder

The second obsessional problem is 'obsessive–compulsive disorder'. This condition is recognized by the presence of certain symptoms, rather than personality traits. It is regarded as an anxiety problem although not everyone with this disorder reports feeling anxious (see Chapter 2).

Until recently obsessive–compulsive disorder was regarded as relatively rare, but it became apparent that its occurrence in the general population was vastly underestimated. It has now been suggested that as many as five million people suffer from the problem in the United States. If the prevalence rates of the disorder are similar in the United Kingdom, then it is possible that as many as one million people suffer from the problem here. Academic research is now showing that obsessional symptoms are quite common in people who don't recognize their obsessional behaviour as problematic.

Furthermore, they are often able to cope at home and at work by developing sophisticated routines which allow them to hide their symptoms. It is only when psychologists and psychiatrists go out into the community that the true picture emerges, as rarely do sufferers complain to their GP.

Symptoms

It is now widely recognized that obsessional symptoms are not rare, but extremely common, up to twice as common as other anxiety disorders such as panic, for example. In addition, many individuals who have been diagnosed as depressed or anxious also suffer from obsessional symptoms. What then, are the symptoms of obsessive–compulsive disorder? As the name indicates, it has a dual character with both obsessional and compulsive components.

An obsession is a recurrent idea, thought, impulse or image, which is experienced, at least initially, as intrusive, unacceptable, or frightening. A compulsion, is a behaviour performed in order to reduce discomfort caused by the obsession. Sometimes, the behaviour is completely irrational, and resembles a superstitious ritual. Other kinds of compulsions are related more logically to the obsession, but are clearly excessive.

Most obsessionals recognize that their disturbing thoughts come from their own mind, and they also recognize that their compulsive behaviours are excessive or unreasonable. In spite of this insight, they feel unable to control their thoughts, or change their behaviour.

The compulsive component of obsessive–compulsive disorder may not be a particular activity that other people can see, were they to be watching. An unacceptable thought might be 'made right' by a purely mental ritual. These 'cognitive' rituals may involve conjuring up a corrective image, or thinking a phrase which somehow 'neutralizes' the unacceptable thought. Counting, or repeating a particular sequence of numbers are also common forms of mental compulsion.

> Jane has problems with obsessional thoughts and images. These are often of a sexual nature, and Jane finds them totally unacceptable. When they come into her mind, she can't seem to concentrate on anything else. They distract her from her work, and they are usually accompanied by feelings of guilt. In order to cope with them, she will try to conjure up what she describes as 'cleansing images'. These are usually linked by a religious theme. Although she feels some relief after conjuring her cleansing images, they are not always sufficient. They have also become more and more complicated, in order to achieve the same sense of relief. Although Jane is happily married, she is unable to talk to her husband about her problem. She feels certain that he will think badly of her. At worst, she expects rejection. Recently, she has become more and more depressed about her thoughts. She has begun to see herself as a 'bad' person, and believes that by having these thoughts, she is betraying her husband. She also feels that if things continue as they are, she will not be able to attend her local church; she believes that she has no rightful place in the congregation if such shameful thoughts cannot be removed.

The purpose of most compulsions, either observable or unobservable, appears to be to reduce the discomfort engendered by obsessional thoughts; however, in some cases, obsessional thoughts can appear in the absence of specific compulsions. These so called 'pure obsessions' are, on occasion, associated with more subtle ways of reducing anxiety – like seeking reassurance from others, for example. People who suffer from these exaggerated concerns are sometimes called 'ruminators'. Another kind of obsessional problem, again, often found in the absence of compulsions, has been termed 'morbid preoccupation'. Morbid preoccupations are similar to obsessions, in that they are upsetting and difficult to control; however, they are usually more realistic than obsessions and are not considered absurd or irrational by the person who experiences them. In many ways, they resemble excessive and persistent worry.

Types of obsessive–compulsive disorder

Washing

'Washers' are characteristically concerned about contaminating themselves or others. As a result, they tend to avoid things or places where they feel contamination is likely. If, as is often the case, they believe that contamination has occurred, then they feel compelled to wash; however this washing is unlike normal washing.

An obsessional will wash over and over again, until absolutely sure that the 'contaminant' has been removed. This can mean being trapped at the sink or washbasin for anything between five minutes and an hour. In severe cases, an obsessional washer will continue until his or her hands bleed. For some, the problem is so severe, that they are unable to leave the sink at all. Washing has been known to continue at the expense of eating and sleeping, until the sufferer collapses, totally exhausted. Contamination fears can also cause enormous domestic problems. An obsessional mother might not be able to cuddle her child, or sustain a normal sexual relationship with her husband.

Roy has had contamination fears for as long as he can remember. Even when he was a child, the thought of getting his hands dirty made him feel uncomfortable. He can recall feeling happier when wearing gloves. As an adult, the thought of contamination still causes him enormous distress. For Roy, the world is a very dangerous place. Simple, everyday activities, have become linked with cleaning rituals. When he gets to work, he must immediately wash his hands; however, to wash his hands, he must go into the toilet – yet another possible source of infection. When Roy gets to the sink, he does not allow himself to touch the taps. He places a paper towel over the tap, and turns it slowly, being very careful not to make contact. He then washes his hands thoroughly. This might take up to 10 minutes on a bad day. While he is washing, he is extremely anxious. If someone comes in, it will be embarrassing. Further, they might disturb his concentration. If the wash is not thorough, he knows that he will have to return, and start all over again. Most days, Roy will wash his hands about fifty times. He loses an average of three hours out of every day, just washing. His hands are sore and cracked, because all the natural protective oils in his skin have been broken down by excessive contact with water and use of strong detergents. He does not believe he will be able to remain in employment for very much longer. Each day is a terrible struggle. Concentration is ruined by unexpected contact with contaminants, and the necessity to plan visits to the toilet without being observed.

Checking

'Checkers', like washers, cannot seem to stop their particular obsessive activity. A 'checker' may need to check things several times before being satisfied that everything is all right. The most common items checked are doors, taps, appliances and light switches. As with washing, the problem can be mildly debilitating to totally incapacitating.

Some individuals feel the need to check so strongly, that they cannot live an ordinary life. Leaving the house can take hours. Each light switch, tap, and door may require up to 300 checks. In order to get to work, the obsessional checker may have to get up extremely early, so as to allow enough time for the checking rituals to be completed.

In addition to this kind of checking behaviour, there is another which is even more difficult to reconcile with a normal life. This involves retracing one's footsteps, or going back to a particular place, to see if one was responsible for doing harm to others. Although most checkers who exhibit this kind of behaviour can see that this is irrational, they find it almost impossible to stop going back. Clearly, such behaviour can have an enormous impact on day-to-day living, as well as prompting doubt about one's sanity, and incurring the dismay of relatives and friends, should they find out.

Bill has checking rituals; he checks most things. However, checking that his car is roadworthy can be particularly problematic. After establishing that the coolant in the radiator is the right level, he replaces the cap. He then turns the cap against the stop up to twenty-five times. Even after twenty-five minor checks of this kind, he can still feel that the cap is not secure. When this happens, Bill will remove the cap, and start again. Once he is satisfied, he then checks the oil. While checking the oil, he often begins to doubt that the radiator cap is firmly on after all. This means that whole procedure must be repeated again. A similar series of checking rituals are associated with the windscreen water bottle, and the engine oil filter cap. On average, getting started can take up to 20 minutes. By this time, Bill feels tense, poorly, and quite down. When he starts driving he is usually distressed and upset.

Other obsessional behaviours

In addition to checking and washing, a number of other obsessional behaviours have been noted. These include a need for symmetry, order, or exactness. Failure to do things in a certain way might lead to extreme discomfort requiring some kind of corrective activity. Obsessional individuals may undertake a particular task, and because of some small error – or disturbing thought – feel compelled to abandon what has been completed, and start all over again. This kind of problem may be related to something called 'primary obsessional slowness', which involves the execution of everyday tasks (like tooth-brushing and shaving) at an extremely slow rate. The root of this problem seems to be a desire to do things in a meticulous way, to a very high standard. Finally, another variant of obsessional behaviour is hoarding. This is a close relative of some of the unusual collecting interests described earlier. The individual feels compelled to collect and store certain objects. These may have no intrinsic value, for example empty tin cans.

These behaviours are dealt with in more detail in Chapter 8.

The main types of obsessional problem are listed in Table 1. The problem with this kind of list is that it implies that the different manifestations are mutually exclusive. This is not the case. It is possible to have several different obsessional complaints at the same time. It is also possible to experience different obsessional complaints at different times. So one could, for example, develop washing and checking compulsions concurrently, or, experience washing compulsions for two years, which then disappear in favour of checking compulsions.

Summary

1. There are a number of normal behaviours, which have an obsessional quality: collecting things, falling in love, and driving ambition, are typical examples. However, these are not necessarily part of a clinical problem.
2. When psychologists and psychiatrists refer to obsessionality,

Table 1: Manifestations of Obsessionality

Obsessive–compulsive personality disorder

1. Perfectionism
2. Preoccupation with detail
3. Insistence on doing things in a particular way
4. Devotion to work
5. Indecisiveness
6. Overconscientiousness
7. Difficulty expressing a range of emotions
8. Lack of generosity
9. Inability to discard possessions

Obsessive–compulsive disorder

Common examples:
1. Washing and cleaning
2. Checking

Less common:
1. Primary obsessional slowness
2. Rituals to do with symmetry and order
3. Hoarding
4. Pure obsessions
5. Morbid preoccupations

---

they are usually referring to one of two diagnosable problems: obsessive–compulsive personality disorder, or obsessive–compulsive disorder.
3. Obsessive–compulsive personality disorder consists of a group of personality traits that tend to cluster together. Broadly speaking, they reflect a tendency to be perfectionist and to show inflexible attitudes. The treatment of obsessive–compulsive personality disorder is best undertaken with a therapist.
4. Obsessive–compulsive disorder can be recognized according to the presence of certain symptoms, rather than character traits. Common examples of obsessive–compulsive disorder are excessive washing and excessive checking. These behaviours are

usually undertaken in response to distressing thoughts. Less common examples of obsessive–compulsive disorder are primary obsessional slowness, a need for symmetry, and hoarding. Unlike obsessive–compulsive personality disorder, obsessive–compulsive disorder is amenable to self-help.

5. Although the obsessive–compulsive personality disorder and obsessive–compulsive disorder are seen diagnostically as separate problems, there appears to be some overlap. Selected obsessional personality traits might be amenable to self-help.

2

Anxiety Problems: How They Start and How They Can be Overcome

Anxiety is an emotional state characterized by changes in one's body, thoughts and behaviour. It tends to be associated with certain things or situations, and most people who are anxious believe that staying in feared situations will result in their anxiety reaching intolerable levels for an indefinite period of time. However, as we shall see, this is not the case, and all the evidence of researchers and health care professionals show that, in fact, anxiety has a limit and can only reach a certain level. Once it reaches this level, it will stay there for a while and then start to come down. Unfortunately, though, most anxious people never find this out because they avoid upsetting the situations to start with.

In this chapter we are going to look quite closely at anxiety problems: how they start, how they go on being problems, and how you can tackle them.

The nature of anxiety

Anxiety is a broad term, and it is helpful to break it down into component parts. There are three parts to the feeling of being anxious:

1. *Physical changes* There are many of these but the most common are: shortness of breath, dizziness, increased heart rate, trembling, muscle tension, sweating, numbness, tingling sensations, dry mouth, abdominal discomfort and nausea.
2. *Thoughts* Different anxiety problems are associated with different anxious thoughts. For example, someone who's afraid of social situations might think 'I'm being watched', whereas somebody experiencing panic might think 'I'm having a heart attack'. In general, anxious thoughts are about being in some kind of danger, or putting others at risk.

3. *Behaviour* Behaviour refers to what you actually do – in this case, when you are anxious. We have already mentioned the most important anxiety-related behaviour, which is avoidance. There are many forms of avoidance: for example, not going into certain situations, or getting out of a situation as soon as possible. However, avoidance behaviour can also be very subtle. An individual might perform a particular action, because he or she believes that performing that action will reduce the chances of something untoward happening. The action in question might have a superstitious quality. The notion that 'touching wood' will somehow help us to avoid a future accident or mishap is a common example.

When trying to overcome anxiety, it is important that all three components – physical symptoms, thoughts, and behaviour – are considered. Later in this book, we will see how relaxation can be used to control physical symptoms (see Chapter 4), and how upsetting thoughts can be modified (see Chapter 5, 9 and 11). Methods allowing you to overcome avoidance behaviour will also be explained (see Chapter 4).

How anxiety problems start

Most health care professionals, like psychologists, would agree that anxiety problems seem to arise because of a combination of predisposing factors and life experiences. In the same way that you inherit eye or hair colour, you might also inherit a predisposition to develop anxiety problems. Presumably this has some kind of biological basis; however, just because your parents are anxious, it doesn't mean that you will be anxious too. Similarly, if you are anxious, this doesn't mean that your children will have the same problem.

In psychological jargon, the total of an individual's life experience is called 'learning history'. When considering the development of psychological problems, we must also take into account what any individual has lived through. Some fears can be traced back to a particular unpleasant event – someone who is afraid of lifts for example, may once have been trapped in a lift. It's also possible to develop fears (phobias) in childhood by watching one's parents. Children often learn about the world by watching the way their parents, or other significant people, react to certain situations. If your father ran out of the room whenever he saw a spider, you may have formed the impression that spiders are extremely dangerous creatures. This kind of learning is called 'modelling'; the learned behaviour is modelled on the actions of another person. As with inheriting certain predispositions, we cannot say for certain that just because a child watches his or her parent being afraid, he or she will also develop the same phobia; parental behaviour is simply another factor to take into consideration.

In summary, there are no direct links between predisposition, learning history, and the development of anxiety disorders. Nevertheless, biological heritage, unpleasant experiences and anxious parents, are all factors which may contribute. Taken together, the presence of each will increase the likelihood of an anxiety disorder developing.

How are anxiety problems maintained?

The notion that fears (or 'phobias') are learned – by either watching models or by experiencing unpleasant events – is largely accepted by a group of psychologists called behaviourists. The original behaviourists believed that phobias are the result of a bad learning experience during which something relatively harmless became associated with something unpleasant. Because of this association, the relatively harmless object, or place, then becomes capable of evoking fear on its own. Furthermore, fear may *generalize*, so that other harmless objects or places are capable of evoking fear. Usually, fear 'spreads' when objects and places share common features. For example, somebody who was trapped in a lift at work, might then become frightened of all lifts. In addition, this fear of lifts may generalize to any small room without windows.

The experience of fear is clearly very unpleasant. Once a person has developed a phobia, he or she is likely to avoid the object or place associated with fear. Approaching a feared object or situation will result in increased anxiety, whereas withdrawal will result in decreased anxiety. It is this, the experience of relief, that makes avoidance more likely in the future. If you find that whenever you get a headache, lying down for five minutes reliably gets rid of it, then you are likely to continue using this particular way of coping. Any behaviour which reduces unpleasant feelings becomes more likely. So, for someone with an anxiety problem, escaping or avoiding places associated with fear becomes the preferred way of coping. Although this strategy is useful in the short term, in the long term, it is most unhelpful because the person never confronts the feared situation, and never has the opportunity to learn that there is nothing to be frightened of. In this way, *avoidance maintains fear.*

What actually happens in anxious situations

If you asked an anxious person, 'What do you think would happen if you stayed in a situation that makes you feel anxious?', s/he might answer any of the following:

> I don't really know, but I expect that my anxiety would get worse and worse.

> I couldn't say, but I guess that my anxiety would get really bad, and it would just stay like that.

> I don't want to think about what would happen. I'd probably go crazy.

The fact is, none of these things would happen. Psychologists know from a number of experiments, as well as from treating patients, that the anxiety response takes a particular form. If an anxious person enters a feared situation, the anxiety will begin to get worse. Usually, when the anxiety reaches a certain point, the person leaves the situation and experiences the relief described earlier. However, if the person stayed in that situation, then s/he would find that, after a certain amount of time, the anxiety would begin to decrease. This reduction in anxiety *has* to happen because our bodies are built that way; anxiety cannot go on getting worse and worse. It reaches a maximum level, and then it begins to go down. But most anxious people never find this out because they avoid the upsetting situations from the beginning.

On the first occasion that an anxious person stays in (is 'exposed' to) a feared situation, her/his anxiety levels may go up, and stay up for quite a long time. In some cases high levels of anxiety can last for several hours. Nevertheless, persistence is the key and is usually rewarded with a gradual reduction in anxiety. On the first 'exposure', this gradual reduction in anxiety may be slow.

On the second exposure, anxiety may again rise, but might not reach the previous highest level. The person may continue to feel anxious for a while, but not for as long as the first time. Anxiety may begin to go down a little earlier than before, and the drop will not take as long.

With each subsequent attempt to stay in the feared situation, anxiety becomes less and less of a problem – because of 'habituation', the situation is no longer so anxiety-provoking because you are getting 'used to it'.

'Exposure' as treatment

Encouraging anxious people to enter and stay in the situations that they fear is a standard behavioural technique, and is commonly referred to as 'exposure therapy'. It is *very* effective, and numerous studies have been conducted demonstrating that continuous exposure to feared situations often results in the long term reduction of anxiety.

Understandably, many people who suffer from anxiety get quite worried when they hear about 'exposure therapy'. They often think it involves being thrown into situations that are quite terrifying. This isn't the case. Later on in the book we will be discussing how a treatment plan can be designed in which discomfort is kept to an absolute minimum (see Chapter 4). So, don't worry!

However, it is impossible to say how long it will take for your anxiety to go down because everybody is different. In general, anxiety may continue to rise for about 15 or 20 minutes. Once it reaches a maximum level, it may stay at that maximum level anywhere between five minutes and half-an-hour.

The anxiety disorders

Obsessive–compulsive disorder is one of several anxiety problems known as the 'anxiety disorders'. However, there is some debate as to whether it should be placed among this group of problems as often people suffering from obsessive–compulsive disorder describe their emotional state without reference to anxiety; they may report feelings of sadness, worry, guilt, and general discomfort, without saying that they are anxious. Here, and in other chapters, the word 'anxiety' will be used as a general term to describe all unpleasant emotional states associated with obsessional symptoms. The term may not correspond exactly with how you feel, but this should not matter too much with respect to treatment.

The anxiety disorders are a group of problems which, although quite different in terms of presenting symptoms, tend to share the same emotional 'flavour'. Fear and excessive worry are common features.

Panic disorder

'Panic disorder' is characterized by the sudden and unexpected onset of a panic attack when the individual experiences a number of frightening symptoms, such as palpitations, dizziness, flushes, and difficulty with breathing. These may be accompanied by thoughts about dying or going mad. This problem is closely associated with another, 'agoraphobia'.

Agoraphobia

Here, the sufferer is frightened of being in places from which escape is difficult or embarrassing in the event of a panic attack. As a result of this, the sufferer will avoid 'agoraphobic situations' – such as being outside his home alone, being in a crowd, or being on a bus or train. Although the relationship between panic and agoraphobia is a strong one, it is also possible to be agoraphobic, without ever having experienced a panic attack.

Agoraphobia, is, as its name suggests, a 'phobic' problem. Phobias are persistent, and often irrational fears, which are associated with particular things or places. Simple phobias are fairly common: a fear of spiders, closed spaces, or flying, for example.

Social phobia

This is a persistent fear of social situations, accompanied by worry about doing something humiliating or embarrassing. As a result of these worries, the social phobic may be reluctant to talk in front of others. He or she may begin to shake when asked to write a cheque, or experience difficulty swallowing food when eating with others. Simple phobics and social phobics tend to avoid situations that are likely to trigger their fears.

Generalized anxiety disorder

Generalized anxiety disorder (or GAD) is characterized by excessive, and often unrealistic, worrying. The afflicted person tends to worry continually about everyday problems – paying bills, holding down a job, or family matters. In addition to worrying excessively, the individual may feel very tense, and have difficulty with getting to sleep.

Post-traumatic stress disorder

A recent addition to the anxiety disorders group is post-traumatic stress disorder (or PTSD). This occurs after an individual has experienced an unusual event, often of a life-threatening nature – for example, being in a crash. The sufferer may have recurrent nightmares or images about the event, be continuously 'on edge', and avoid anything associated with the distressing event. In some cases, additional problems of a more complex nature develop, such as, depression, being unable to plan for the future, difficulty relating to others, drinking too much, and feeling 'guilty' about surviving (especially if friends or relatives lost their lives).

In many ways, diagnostic systems are misleading. They give the impression that people with anxiety problems can be neatly slotted under different headings. In practice, this is not the case. It is often extremely difficult to say exactly what problem someone has. Although an individual's main problem may be obsessive–compulsive disorder, s/he may also have had the occasional panic attack; someone with a fear of social situations might also worry a great deal. The above summaries are given only as a rough guide to the sort of problems associated with anxiety. If you feel that as well as having an obsessional problem, you also have other anxiety problems, it might be worth finding out more. A reading list is supplied at the end of this book.

Treating anxiety disorders

As mentioned earlier, avoidance perpetuates anxiety, and so encouraging people with anxiety problems to enter and stay in their feared situation(s) has become a standard and effective treatment technique. It is based on the results of studies which show that repeated exposure to feared situations can result in the long-term reduction of anxiety.

'Exposure therapy' for obsessive–compulsive disorder

The general principles of anxiety maintenance and reduction, can also give us some insight into how obsessive–compulsive disorder symptoms are maintained, and how they might be treated. Lets take the two most common obsessional symptoms – washing and checking – as examples.

Compulsive washing, might be considered the result of having a sort of 'dirt' or 'germ' phobia. The individual is frightened by the thought of contamination. Subsequently, he or she will avoid certain things and places considered to be contaminated – public lavatories, for example. If contact with a contaminant is unavoidable, the individual will become extremely anxious. Relief is achieved by sustained and repeated washing. In effect, washing is another type of avoidance behaviour; through washing, the likelihood of infection is reduced, and anxiety diminishes, temporarily. However, prolonged exposure to contamination will result in anxiety reduction through the process of habituation i.e. you get used to it. After anxiety reduction has occurred, the urge to wash will be less intense, as it is no longer necessary as a means of reducing anxiety.

With compulsive checking, the individual might fear being responsible for harming others or causing accidents. An accident might occur, for example, as a result of leaving the cooker switched on. Irrational doubts about whether or not the cooker is still on results in high levels of anxiety or discomfort. The only way of reducing this discomfort is to check the cooker. After checking the cooker several times, the individual may experience a sense of relief. The checking behaviour is therefore another method of avoiding imaginary catastrophes, and of reducing anxiety. By confronting situations usually associated with checking, the individual finds that discomfort eventually subsides. This, in turn, of course, reduces the necessity to check.

The standard behavioural treatment of obsessive–compulsive disorder involves exposing the individual to feared situations. This is usually accompanied by directions to resist urges to wash and check. The resistance of urges can be regarded as a second component of treatment, and this will be discussed fully in Chapter 4.

Summary

1. Anxiety problems develop as a result of predisposing factors, learning history or a combination of the two.
2. Anxiety is often maintained by avoidance: by avoiding certain situations, anxious individuals never learn that the feared consequences they expect rarely happen.
3. When anxious people enter feared situations, they usually

experience an increase in anxiety. If they remain in the feared situation, anxiety levels usually drop.

4. Behaviour therapists encourage their patients to stay in feared situations until anxiety levels drop to tolerable levels. This form of treatment has proved very effective with all of the anxiety disorders.

5. Obsessive–compulsive disorder is a member of the anxiety disorders. Although many individuals with obsessive–compulsive disorder feel that anxiety isn't a very good description of how they feel, the term 'anxiety' can still be used to describe the general discomfort associated with obsessionality.

3

The Development of Obsessions and Compulsions, and How to Assess Your Symptoms

Unlike the other anxiety disorders, obsessive–compulsive disorder has more variants. However, it does appear to conform to a basic pattern: a mental event, or an assessment of a particular situation, produces discomfort or anxiety; this is then reduced by a behaviour. This is not always the case, and an individual may be able to reduce discomfort by performing a mental ritual or seeking reassurance. In this chapter, we will be taking a closer look at obsessive–compulsive disorder, whilst providing a framework within which you can make sense of your symptoms.

The development of obsessions

Thought suppression

Obsessions are usually intrusive, repetitive, largely unwanted, and very difficult to control. Unlike most thoughts, obsessions cannot be ignored. Obsessions can be a single word, a phrase or a sentence. They can also take the form of upsetting images. In some cases, the obsession takes the form of thoughts *and* images. When an obsession first occurs, it is usually regarded as unacceptable. For example, a religious person may have a blasphemous thought, or a doting parent might have an image of killing his or her child. Because the thought is unacceptable, or alien, the individual may try to suppress, or block it. Although this is a natural response, evidence suggests that suppressing any thought results in its more frequent return. This is easily demonstrated: try to *not* think of a chair. Close your eyes, and try it for a few minutes. What happened? In all likelihood you kept on thinking of chairs! Logically, every time you try to stop thinking of something, you have to represent it in your mind first.

Some obsessions are troublesome, not because they are morally unacceptable, but because they are nonsensical. An individual might be bothered by a particular phrase such as '. . . and then there were three'. The inability to dismiss the thought eventually becomes distressing, and its persistence interferes with concentration and tasks undertaken as part of everyday life.

Odd thoughts are normal

Once upon a time, persistent and disturbing thoughts were considered peculiar to obsessional patients. However, in the 1970s and 1980s, research showed that most people experience this kind of thought. Here are a few examples of what are termed 'normal obsessions' – normal, because they were volunteered by ordinary people with no psychiatric history:

- I'm going to hit someone
- I'm going to jump in front of the train
- I'm going to rape my girlfriend
- I'm going to swear out aloud in church
- I hope my partner dies
- I'm going to strangle my kitten

Many of these 'obsessions' are about unacceptable behaviour; thoughts or impulses to do with blasphemy, sexual acts, and violence. Their occurrence may cause a certain amount of distress or dismay ('Where did that come from?'); however, they are usually not given special significance. It is only when these thoughts are given special significance, or considered meaningful, that an obsessional problem might develop. Consider the following example.

> Lucy was a young mother with a beautiful two-year-old son, David. She was perfectly happy, and doted on him. One afternoon, she was preparing dinner, cutting vegetables with a large knife. David was playing on the floor behind her. Suddenly, out of nowhere, she thought to herself: I could stab my son. She was very disturbed by this thought, and she resolved not to think it again. In doing so, she was immediately aware of the thought again. Every time she tried not to think it, the thought came back. She then reprimanded herself for having the thought in the first place: 'I must be mad to have had that thought'. This made her quite worried, and she began to feel very anxious. She remembered reading once, how a perfectly respectable mother had suddenly gone mad, and killed members of her family. Lucy

then began to ruminate: 'It can't be right to have a thought like that. There must be something wrong with me. What if I did go mad? What if I suddenly turned around and killed David?' She placed the knife in a drawer, closed it, and decided to take a break. When she went back to the drawer, it reminded her of the thought: I could stab my son. At this point, she began thinking, 'There really is something wrong with me'.

In the above example, we can see how a random, distressing thought, is given special significance. The way we respond to our random intrusive thoughts determines whether they become a problem or not. Suppressing a thought may give it special significance. Also, worrying about it can have the same effect. It is perhaps ironic that the people least likely to do harm to others are those who worry about doing harm the most when they have a distressing thought! It is because they find the idea of thinking such things so unacceptable, that they experience high levels of discomfort. In an attempt to reduce these high levels of discomfort, they may develop compulsive behaviours.

When considering the process by which random upsetting thoughts become obsessions, it is clear that the response to an upsetting thought is more important than the thought itself. The evaluation of an upsetting thought is strictly termed 'appraisal', and the type of appraisal made of a particular thought will depend on the kind of person making it. A thought is more likely to be determined as unacceptable if an individual has high personal standards, or is very conscientious. This account would seem to favour those theories of obsessive–compulsive disorder which posit a predisposing obsessional personality. Another implication of this account is that obsessions need not always start off as unpleasant thoughts. For example, a pleasant sexual day-dream might develop beyond the point of personal acceptability. This negative appraisal might lead to guilt and attempts to suppress the thought. Fears related to being 'found out' may then lead to compulsive behaviours.

Underlying beliefs

Another factor to take into account when considering the development of obsessional problems is underlying beliefs. We all have particular beliefs about ourselves and the world around us. Presumably, these are formed as a result of our learning history.

It is possible that people who find certain thoughts extremely distressing have quite rigid beliefs about their significance. It is also possible that these beliefs have developed subsequent to a particular experience. Consider the following:

Mary was an obsessional patient who constantly had to check that she had not done any harm to anyone. She would have the thought 'I think I've caused an accident', and then have to retrace her steps. It was as though she had an underlying belief that thinking something was the same as doing something. The anxiety which she felt after thinking about harming others seemed to be just as high as the anxiety she might have felt if she had actually committed some kind of harmful act. Where did that belief come from? When questioned in therapy, she remembered a particular incident that she had experienced as a child. She had an uncle whom she disliked immensely. Sometimes the uncle got drunk, and taunted her cruelly. One night, she prayed that the uncle would die. The following day, her mother told her that her uncle had died of a heart attack. Mary assumed that she was responsible.

From this example we can see how a particular belief might be formed. However, it might not have its effect for some time. Often, a basic belief or assumption can be dormant until a similar event 'activates' it. Mary's early belief was reactivated when, as an adult, she wished her boss was dead! Shortly after, her boss had an accident. It was soon after this that her obsessional checking started.

The development of compulsions

Rules and rituals

The purpose of compulsions is to reduce anxiety or discomfort. Compulsions are repetitive, and under the individual's control. They are different from obsessions in this respect. Obsessions are perceived as being out of control, or at best, very difficult to control. Although washing and checking are the most common compulsions, there are many others. In addition, even common washing and checking compulsions may need to be executed in a particular way; that is, according to rather idiosyncratic rules. These rules are often to ensure the compulsion is effective.

William was a compulsive washer. After going to the toilet, he felt that his hands were contaminated, and if not washed thoroughly, would remain contaminated. He was worried that he might leave his germs on door handles and anything else he might touch. He had intrusive thoughts about people suffering from diseases which he was personally responsible for spreading. At first, several hand washes were enough to reduce his anxiety; however, he began to feel that simply washing his hands was not enough. His hands had to be washed in a particular way. He had to rub his palms together first, then lock his fingers together, while continuing to rub. He then had to place his right hand under the tap, and rotate it. It was necessary to repeat this procedure with his left hand. If he got this sequence wrong, he still felt unclean. He would then have to go right back to the beginning, and start all over again.

It is impossible to say why William chose to wash his hands in this way. When asked, he couldn't really give an answer. It just felt better, if washing was always performed according to this particular sequence. Perhaps this is not so surprising. If we want to do something well, we will try to do it systematically. If, for example, you believe that failure to wash your hands correctly might result in other people suffering, then you are likely to take extra care that washing is effective. Developing a systematic way of washing is a plausible method of ensuring an effective wash.

The relationship between contamination and washing makes sense because washing really does remove germs. Some obsessive–compulsive disorder sufferers develop rituals which reduce anxiety, but these rituals are only remotely related to the obsessional thoughts – for example: responding to an intrusive thought about family members being involved in an accident by turning around three times. Again, this kind of behaviour seems odd at first sight, but is it really that odd? Most people have some sort of superstitious behaviour that, when performed, reduces anxiety: many students take lucky charms into the examination room; a particular pen may be associated with exam success, and used in every exam thereafter; people still throw salt over their shoulders, and touch wood to avoid calamities. Because calamities are rare, superstitious behaviours seem pretty effective. If performed regularly, the individual (usually) never finds out that the disasters that superstitious behaviours are meant to prevent never happen anyway.

Sometimes, anxiety-reducing rituals occur only in the mind. They serve the same function as behavioural rituals, but are less embarrassing because they can't be seen by others. Because they are more secret, they are often called 'covert rituals'. Consider the following:

Henry had an obsessional image of harming his girlfriend. When this image occurred, he had to conjure another to 'make things right' or cancel the first image. This involved imagining a photograph of his girlfriend, an ivory crucifix, and a particular painting of Jesus Christ, in that order. After performing this covert ritual, Henry would feel greatly relieved.

Most obsessive–compulsive disorder sufferers recognize that their compulsions are irrational. As a result, compulsions are often resisted. That is, the individual tries to stop him- or herself performing the compulsive behaviour. This leads to a build-up of tension, which is reduced when the behaviour is performed; however, it is sometimes the case that after some time, the individual stops resisting the compulsion, and performs it automatically. Some individuals, on the other hand, perform compulsions automatically right from the start.

Reassurance seeking and avoidance

People with obsessional problems often ask for reassurance. This is especially the case during treatment. When asked to perform a particular task, the obsessional patient might say something like: 'I know I've got to do this to get better, but no harm will come to anybody as a result, will it?'. It is very tempting for a therapist, under such circumstances to reply 'Of course not!'. But this kind of reassurance can be largely unhelpful. This is because reassurance often serves the same function as avoidance. If you ask someone for reassurance, and they give it to you, you are allowing them to share responsibility for your own actions. This reduces discomfort and anxiety. But as was suggested earlier, it is important to confront feared situations and wait for anxiety to rise, and subsequently subside. In obsessive–compulsive disorder, asking for reassurance is simply a subtle method of side-stepping full responsibility, and of avoiding the anxiety that a particular activity provokes. We will consider ways of dealing with reassurance seeking later in the book (see Chapter 5).

Assessing your problem

We have already said that obsessive–compulsive disorder is somewhat different to the other anxiety disorders, because of its complexity. It is associated with a wider group of symptoms, which can be mental, behavioural, or both. If you want to treat your obsessive–compulsive disorder symptoms, then you need to have a good understanding of what they are, and how they fit together.

First of all, you need to get a rough idea of what your problem 'looks like'. You might be feeling a little uncertain about how the preceding information relates to your symptoms; you might be unsure about whether you have obsessive–compulsive disorder at all! So, let's take a closer look at your symptoms. Try ticking the boxes shown below, in answer to the listed questions.

Avoidance
Do you avoid going to certain places or
   situations because you fear they will
   trigger unwanted thoughts or result in
   compulsive behaviour?   Yes ☐ No ☐

Obsessions
Do you have persistent unwanted thoughts? Yes ☐ No ☐
Do you have persistent unwanted images?   Yes ☐ No ☐
Are these mental events unacceptable to you? Yes ☐ No ☐
Are these mental events nonsensical
   or bizarre?   Yes ☐ No ☐

Discomfort
When you get unwanted thoughts or images,
   do you feel anxiety/discomfort?   Yes ☐ No ☐

Compulsions
Do you sometimes feel an urge to do
   certain things?   Yes ☐ No ☐
Do you eventually 'give in' to the urge?   Yes ☐ No ☐
Is the compulsion visible (i.e. someone
   watching could notice)?   Yes ☐ No ☐

Is the compulsion invisible (i.e. it
happens in your mind)?   Yes ☐   No ☐

Discomfort reduction
When you perform your compulsion does
your anxiety/discomfort decrease?   Yes ☐   No ☐
Do you sometimes ask people for an opinion
about something you did, or didn't do, in
the hope that they will say something
reassuring?   Yes ☐   No ☐

After considering the above questions, you may find that you have
ticked several boxes, or only a few. That doesn't matter too much at
this stage. The purpose of this exercise is to see how your symptoms
correspond with the usual features of obsessive–compulsive disorder and to note the general form of your problem. You may find
that your symptoms are not typical: perhaps you get unwanted
thoughts, but don't have any compulsions; on the other hand you
might feel that you are compulsive, but don't have any obsessions.
Although this is sometimes the case, most obsessive–compulsive
disorder sufferers get both. A common mistake is a failure to
recognize covert rituals as compulsions. As suggested earlier
compulsions can be undertaken in the mind. If you have been
performing covert rituals for some time, they might occur so swiftly
that you hardly notice them any more. If, on the other hand, you
genuinely get obsessional thoughts in the absence of any compulsive
symptoms, you might be what is often termed, a 'pure obsessional',
or ruminator. Pure obsessions, will be considered in greater detail
later in the book (see Chapter 9).

If you found completing the assessment exercise helped you to
make some sense of your symptoms, or at least made you think
about them in a more systematic way, then you might try looking at
Appendix 1. This is a more detailed version. If you decide
to complete this detailed self-assessment form, then save it for
future comparison. After undertaking your self-help programme,
answer the questions again, and note where improvement has
occurred.

Other compulsion-like behaviours

Before concluding this chapter, a few words should be said about
behaviours which resemble compulsions, but are really something

quite different. If you find that you keep on doing the same thing over and over again, but don't have any idea why, then you should probably see your doctor for a check up. We all, on occasion, do things automatically without thinking; however, the sort of problems referred to here are more extreme, more persistent, and sometimes more embarrassing. For example, being unable to inhibit certain impulses, like swearing in public places. Repetitive behaviours which are rather mechanical, involuntary, and serve no particular function, are comparable to problems like 'nervous tics'. Tics, and persistent involuntary activity, can be associated with neurological problems. These cannot be treated by self-help methods, and medication may be necessary. Your GP will be able to tell you if this is the case, and will refer you to an appropriate specialist.

Summary

1. Most people experience odd, or unusual thoughts. Under normal circumstances, these are dismissed with relative ease.
2. If an unusual thought is considered unacceptable, or is considered to have special meaning, this may result in responses which ultimately strengthen the thought; for example attempts to suppress the thought may lead to its more frequent occurrence.
3. The way an individual appraises an intrusive thought is determined by the sort of person that s/he is, and the beliefs s/he has about her-/himself and the world around.
4. Certain beliefs can be formed as a result of learning experiences.
5. Although the relationship between an obsessional thought and a compulsive behaviour can be logical, this isn't always the case. Some compulsive behaviours have a superstitious quality.
6. When assessing obsessive–compulsive disorder, a number of features should be taken into consideration. These include the presence of obsessional thoughts, compulsive behaviour, avoidance, and reassurance seeking. It is important to make sense of obsessional symptoms within a meaningful framework.
7. Not all repetitive behaviours can be attributed to obsessive–compulsive disorder. Mechanical behaviours that cannot be inhibited and do not relate to any subjective experience might be caused by a neurological problem. Neurological problems cannot be treated using self-help.

4

Exposure Therapy for Obsessive-Compulsive Disorder: Changing the Way You Behave

Having looked at what happens in anxious situations, and having made an assessment of symptoms, we can now turn to the treatment of obsessive–compulsive disorder, but in more detail this time.

It is widely agreed that the most effective treatment for anxiety disorders and obsessive–compulsive disorder involves getting the individual to enter and stay in his/her feared situation(s) as repeated attempts at this – 'exposures' – have been shown to reduce anxiety in the long term. This treatment is called 'exposure therapy'. With this technique is coupled another strategy: encouraging the individual to stop executing the behaviour he/she normally uses to reduce discomfort. This technique is called 'response-prevention', and the whole treatment package referred to as 'exposure and response-prevention'.

How does exposure therapy work?

It is impossible to say exactly how this technique works, although there are a number of explanations. We will consider two of them.

Behaviour modification

Repeated events lose their effect
When entering and staying in anxious situations, there is an increase, and then a decrease in anxiety levels. This happens because the nervous system is built in a particular way. We tend to react to new things, but become less 'reactive' when we get used to them. For example, if you are reading a book at home, and suddenly there is a loud bang, you will probably jump. Your heart rate will go up, and you will start to listen attentively. If it happens again, you will still react, but you might not jump the same way you did the first time. If the banging continues, you will gradually get used to it, and your heart rate will return to its usual

35

speed. This process by which we get accustomed to repeated events, is called 'habituation'. The potential to 'habituate' is a property of the nervous system, and habituation can occur independently of what we are thinking at the time. Exposure therapy may work at a very basic level, and the reduction in anxiety may reflect changes in nervous system activity.

The effect of rewards on behaviour

Escaping from an unpleasant situation will reduce anxiety. This gives the individual a feeling of great relief. We know from experiments that if any behaviour is followed by a reward, that behaviour is more likely to occur again. For example, if you pick up a really good bargain in your local book shop, it is highly likely you will drop in there again. In jargon, the behaviour is said to be 'reinforced'. When an anxious person escapes from an unpleasant situation, the avoidance behaviour is immediately rewarded by a reduction in anxiety levels. This of course, makes avoidance more likely in the future. The avoidance behaviour has therefore been reinforced.

The effect of withdrawing reward on behaviour

If you kept on going to your local book shop, but no longer found any bargains, your behaviour would change. At first, you might still drop in quite frequently; however, very soon, you would only go there as often as you did before you found your bargain. If a particular behaviour stops being reinforced, it will eventually stop or return to initial levels. The jargon term used to describe this process is 'extinction'. If you stay in an unpleasant situation long enough, your anxiety will eventually habituate (i.e. decrease). Therefore, leaving the situation will no longer be associated with anxiety reduction. In other words, your avoidance will not be reinforced by a sense of relief, and you will be less likely to do the same thing in the future. In this way, your avoidance behaviour is extinguished.

How habituation, reinforcement, and extinction relate to the treatment of obsessive–compulsive disorder

These principles are thought to underlie the use of exposure and response prevention with obsessive–compulsive disorder. The obsessive–compulsive disorder individual is encouraged to stay in situations that are perceived as unpleasant until anxiety reduction occurs. In other words, the anxiety habituates. When anxiety goes right down, there is little point performing an anxiety-reducing ritual because it is no longer reinforcing. Performing an anxiety-reducing ritual will no longer be followed by a feeling of relief. The ritual ceases to be 'rewarding', and eventually becomes extinct.

Changing beliefs and expectations

While participating in a behavioural treatment programme, an individual will no doubt experience psychological changes, too. You could say, for example, that as a result of undertaking 'exposure and response-prevention', the individual learns to cope with feared situations, and learns that compulsive rituals serve no useful function. The result of this new learning is that the individual modifies his or her beliefs about what is, and what isn't frightening. In effect, learning to cope with previously feared situations makes the individual 'change his/her mind'. He or she will then start to think about things in a different way.

These psychological changes may occur automatically while participating in an exposure and response-prevention programme. However, some therapists choose to make these psychological changes central to their practice of behaviour therapy: while conducting therapy, they concentrate on trying to persuade patients to think differently about feared situations, and work towards changing the patient's fundamental beliefs. The emphasis is on mental change, rather than on behavioural change alone. Due to this emphasis on thinking and beliefs, this approach has come to be known as 'cognitive–behaviour therapy'. Cognitive refers to thinking and thinking processes.

Behavioural vs cognitive treatment

Although professional opinion differs with regard to the relative merits of a purely behavioural approach compared with a cognitive–behavioural approach, the two approaches are in fact complementary, and marry rather well in practice. In this book, the majority of exercises are behavioural. Nevertheless, some general advice about changing 'thinking style' is also included. The behavioural emphasis is largely due to the fact that cognitive or thinking approaches tend to work better with a therapist present. In therapy, cognitive change is usually achieved by engaging the patient in a kind of debate. Exposure and response-prevention on the other hand, can be undertaken alone. In fact, most behavioural therapy is conducted in the absence of a therapist in the form of homework assignments.

Ways of making exposure therapy easier

If you are an anxious person, then going into situations which make you feel anxious can be extremely difficult. For many people with obsessive–compulsive disorder, the whole idea of exposure is extremely frightening, and even with the support of a therapist it may not be an attractive proposition – however motivated you are. Although tolerating high levels of anxiety can result in quick 'habituation' (see p. 36), this procedure isn't to everyone's liking. If, on your first attempt, you become so anxious that you have a panic attack, then you will probably be less inclined to continue. You might lose confidence, and even abandon the idea of self-help altogether.

For this reason, it's a good idea to undertake exposure to feared situations in stages. Thus, exposure to mildly distressing situations should precede exposure to more distressing situations. This approach is called 'graded exposure'. Before undertaking any exposure at all, you'll have to decide which situations you are going to deal with first. The following instructions are to that end.

First, list situations which make you uncomfortable. Then order the list according to how much anxiety or discomfort you would expect to experience on entering those situations. Rate each situation using the eight-point anxiety scale below.

0	1	2	3	4	5	6	7	8
No anxiety		Slight anxiety		Moderate anxiety		Marked anxiety		Extreme anxiety

Here is a list of situations which may provoke anxiety if you have contamination fears. Each has been rated using the eight-point scale.

Using a public lavatory   8

Walking down a dirty street	2
Using a lavatory at work	7
Using a stranger's pen	3
Using bus seats	4
Using an aeroplane toilet	8
Sleeping in a hotel bed	7
Touching my shoes	2
Touching newspapers	1
Using my own lavatory	3
Emptying the bin	5
Using other people's cutlery	6
Touching a friend's child	8
Sitting in my GP's surgery	6

When you are writing down your list of feared situations, write down as many as you can. You don't need to be selective, just get as many down on paper as you can think of. The more you have, the easier it will be to select an appropriate set for your self-help plan. A few guidelines might be useful at this point. Some people avoid many situations, most of which are quite different. When you put together your graded exposure plan, try to gather items together that are linked by an underlying theme. Clearly, the items above are linked by a fear of contamination. Although it isn't essential that your exposure items are all to do with the same problem, it is more logical. Further, don't include items that you will have no opportunity to practise. For example, putting 'hotel beds' in your plan, when you have no intention of going on holiday, or anywhere near a hotel, isn't very useful.

Once you have all of your items, select between five and ten situations which can be put on an 'anxiety ladder'. Place low-anxiety items at the bottom, moderate-anxiety items in the middle, and high-anxiety items at the top. Also try to make each step go up by roughly the same amount of anxiety.

Here are two examples of six-stage anxiety ladders. The first is practical and systematic, the second impractical and unsystematic.

Anxiety ladder no. 1

Step 6	Using other people's cutlery	6
Step 5	Emptying the dustbin	5
Step 4	Using bus seats	4

Step 3	Using my own lavatory	3
Step 2	Touching my shoes	2
Step 1	Touching newspapers	1

Anxiety ladder no. 2

Step 6	Sleeping in a hotel bed	7
Step 5	Sitting in my GP's surgery	6
Step 4	Emptying the dustbin	5
Step 3	Touching my shoes	2
Step 2	Walking down a dirty street	2
Step 1	Touching newspapers	1

In anxiety ladder no. 1, anxiety ratings are spaced at regular intervals, and all the items are relatively practical. In anxiety ladder no. 2, anxiety ratings are uneven, steps 2 and 3 are the same, and steps 5 and 6 are rather impractical. Always choose items that you can actually do something about.

Of course, it may be the case that your ladder-item ratings do not permit a nice, systematic, practical ladder. In which case, you just have to do your best given these limitations. Nevertheless, with a little imagination and some serious thought, it is usually possible to order items systematically. The technical term used to describe an anxiety ladder is a 'graded hierarchy'.

Once you have constructed your graded hierarchy, you then begin exposing yourself to the first item. Your anxiety will go up a little, and then go down. You may have to put yourself in to this situation several times before significant decreases in anxiety occur. Once you can handle that situation, and only then, should you move up the ladder by one step. In this way, you ensure success, and make the whole business of exposure less upsetting. When you have completed your ladder, construct another one using more challenging items. Again, the same principles apply. Go up a step only after mastering the preceding one.

Relaxation

The above procedure can be modified slightly if you still feel worried about exposure. This can be achieved by practising relaxation, and trying to relax while you expose yourself to anxiety provoking situations. This technique is called 'systematic desentization', and was developed by a psychiatrist, Joseph Wolpe, in the 1950s. The basic idea underlying this approach, is that it is impossible to be anxious and relaxed at the same time; therefore, if you practise relaxation, you might be able to stop becoming anxious as you work up your graded hierarchy of unpleasant situations. In its original form, increasing levels of relaxation were paired with increasingly unpleasant situations: as soon as one step is mastered, you move onto the next; however, if you begin to feel at all anxious, you move back down to the previous step.

There is some debate as to how useful this technique is in its original form as some therapists believe that a little anxiety is necessary to produce therapeutic change. Regardless of the technique's theoretical weaknesses, it can be useful as an intermediate stage. So, if you really feel worried about even the first step on your ladder, you might consider practising relaxation, and then try to relax as you perform your first exposure exercise; however, in the long term, you should probably work towards learning to tolerate mild levels of anxiety.

Learning to relax

Although we use the word relaxation in everyday speech, psychologists use the word to specify a particular procedure. This involves learning to relax various muscle groups all over the body. This is achieved by tensing them first, and then relaxing them. After this has been learned, you are then instructed to relax various parts of your body, without tensing them first. Finally, you are required to get into a relaxed state fairly quickly, by taking a deep breath, holding it for a few moments, and exhaling slowly. While exhaling you usually say the word '*relax*' to yourself. These three types of exercise are called 'deep relaxation', 'quick relaxation', and 'applied relaxation'.

Relaxation tapes There are numerous relaxation tapes currently available. You will probably be able to find one in your local 'health food', or book shop. These usually talk you through the procedures described above. Unfortunately, there are a number of so-called relaxation tapes on the market in which somebody with a particular philosophical view asks you to relax, and then talks about peace or harmony against a background of ethereal sounds. Although this kind of thing is quite pleasant to listen to, it's not what most psychologists have in mind when they refer to relaxation procedures. So, if you do buy a tape, make sure it includes the kind of exercises described above. If you can't find a tape, then you will find the basic relaxation exercises at the back of this book (see Appendix II). It is possible to memorize the exercises and perform them yourself; however, most people find a tape useful, because it sets an appropriate pace and assists concentration.

Practice Remember, relaxation must be practised. Listening to a relaxation tape a few times will not be sufficient to acquire the skill. Most people do not regard relaxation as a skill – preferring instead to think of it as something that just happens when you're not tense. This may be true for some people, but not for everyone. You may be somebody who needs to acquire relaxation skills, and this necessitates practice. Usually, about 25 minutes every day is necessary at the beginning. Deep relaxation is practised for about one or two weeks, before moving on to quick relaxation. As you get better at relaxation, practice sessions can be spread further and further apart. Applied relaxation can be employed in situations which make you tense. It should not be considered as a deep breath and nothing else. It is the complete relaxation of your body within a few seconds. This can only be achieved after hours of practice! Many people who use relaxation tapes as part of their anxiety treatment find them beneficial in a general sense, and carry on using them long after finishing treatment. They usually use them about once a week, or at times when they feel under stress.

Once you have acquired relaxation skills, you can then try step one on your anxiety ladder. Choose a time when you are not stressed and are feeling relatively good. You might prepare for an exposure session by practising some deep, or quick, relaxation exercises first. As you approach the problem situation, begin relaxing. Make sure that you are aware of how anxiety starts for you. It may be a 'knot' in your stomach, a dry mouth, or increased heart rate. Everyone has different early warning signs, although they usually involve some kind of physical change. Try to control your anxiety symptoms at the earliest possible opportunity by using the applied relaxation exercise. Do not let your anxiety get too high, otherwise you might feel that you cannot cope, and leave the situation. Remember, if you are using relaxation, you shouldn't be feeling anxious in the first place.

In all likelihood, you will find it very difficult to relax to the point where you feel no anxiety whatsoever. For this reason, applied relaxation is probably best viewed as a means of 'taking the edge off' of your anxiety if you are finding it difficult to tolerate.

Ways of making response-prevention easier

Many obsessive–compulsive disorder individuals find preventing their usual compulsive behaviours as hard as entering anxiety-provoking situations. However, we can make response prevention easier, in the same way that we made exposure easier – that is, by ordering tasks within a graded hierarchy. For someone with contamination fears, anxiety reduction is accomplished by washing. The idea of contaminating oneself as part of an exposure programme and of not washing at all is unacceptable. Nevertheless, one can delay washing, reduce the amount of time spent washing, or execute both strategies at once.

After contamination the following self-imposed delay, and compulsion-reduction hierarchy could be attempted:

Step 5   Wait for 10 minutes, then wash for   1 minute
Step 4   Wait for   8 minutes, then wash for   3 minutes
Step 3   Wait for   5 minutes, then wash for   5 minutes
Step 2   Wait for   2 minutes, then wash for   8 minute
Step 1   Wait for   1 minute, then wash for 10 minutes

As with the exposure hierarchy, undertake each step in turn, mastering one before going on to the next. Using this kind of plan, the urge to wash follows a similar pattern to anxiety: it tends to rise, then after a while, decreases in intensity. Once you have learned to delay washing for half-an-hour, or an hour, you may not feel the need to wash at all.

Conclusion

Anxiety consists of physical changes, behaviours and upsetting thoughts. Collectively, exposure, response-prevention, and relaxation, might help you to change your behaviour, and moderate the physical changes associated with anxiety. In the next chapter, we will continue to consider how the practice of exposure and response-prevention can be made easier; however the emphasis will be on thinking rather than behavioural and physical aspects.

Summary

1. The preferred treatment for obsessive–compulsive disorder is

exposure and response-prevention. This is a behavioural treatment, in which the individual is encouraged to confront difficult situations, and to refrain from executing compulsive rituals.

2. The effectiveness of this treatment can be explained in several ways: anxiety may be reduced during exposure by the process of habituation; compulsive rituals, which are usually executed in order to reduce anxiety, become redundant once habituation has occurred.

3. Alternatively, the individual may change the way he or she thinks about feared situations, while participating in an exposure and response-prevention programme. In effect, the feared situation is re-evaluated, and no longer considered frightening.

4. Exposure and response-prevention can be made easier by the use of graded hierarchies or anxiety ladders.

5. Relaxation techniques can be used to reduce the unpleasant physical sensations associated with anxiety during exposure.

5

Exposure Therapy for Obsessive–Compulsive Disorder: Changing the Way You Think

Under the right conditions, we can all change the way we think about ourselves. People often talk about giving themselves a 'pep talk' or 'psyching themselves up' when they have to face a problem or some demanding task. They may say things to themselves like: 'You can do it!', 'Go for it!', or 'Keep going!'. They recognize that coaching can be very useful, and that in the absence of a real coach, encouragement has to come from within (or from an imaginary figure). Sports-people will appreciate this point: what a sports-person is saying to him-/herself at a critical point in an event can have a dramatic effect on performance.

Psychologists use a number of techniques to help people change the way they think about themselves – and about the world around them. One of these is 'self-instruction' – a kind of formal way of talking to yourself. You can use this technique to help you get through your treatment exercises. At it's simplest, self-instruction involves rehearsing statements which help you to cope. When you are anxious your head is usually filled with unhelpful statements like: 'I can't stand it any more!', 'I've got to get out of here!', or 'Something terrible is going to happen!'. It's very difficult under such circumstances to think rationally. Therefore, it's useful to prepare 'coping statements', which you can remember – or read on a flash-card – when anxiety threatens.

Coping with a situation can usually be broken down into three stages:

- Preparing to cope
- Dealing with the situation
- How you respond to your performance immediately after.

These different stages will be considered in some detail in this chapter, and suggestions will be made for appropriate self-instruction. The use of pre-prepared statements is also featured.

45

Motivation for change

An important factor in the success of any self-help programme is motivation. Most of this book is about confronting situations which you find upsetting. Although you might be motivated by the idea of overcoming your problems, you probably feel less enthusiastic about entering situations that cause distress! One of the most important first steps in any self-help plan is to make sure that *you* know exactly why *you're* doing it. A clear notion of why you are undertaking your own treatment can be a very useful motivational trigger. To clarify your thoughts, ask yourself the following questions:

- Are there things that I can't do now, that I'll be able to do in the future, once I overcome my problem?
- How will my life be improved on the whole, once I have overcome my problem?

The first question requires specific answers. The second is more general. Try making lists in answer to the questions above. Shown below are typical examples from someone with contamination fears.

Things that I will be able to do:

- Cuddle my children without feeling anxious
- Be more intimate with my husband
- Go out shopping without worrying about using public lavatories
- Go to evening classes
- Accept invitations to dinner without worrying about embarrassing myself.

How will life be improved?

- I won't feel I'm a bad mother
- There will be fewer domestic arguments
- I'll be able to enjoy my family
- I'll have greater personal freedom
- I'll have a social life again
- If I get a qualification, I might be able to work again.

Once you have made your lists, try to remind yourself as often as possible of all the advantages associated with coping. You might even try day-dreaming about the future – imagining yourself doing something you haven't done for a very long time and enjoying it. With enough practice, you will be able to conjure up a positive picture of yourself with less effort.

If you remind yourself in this way:

- You could feel more motivated to begin your exercises
- You might make a strong link between a positive image of yourself and undertaking your exercises
- You might begin to look forward to your exercises
- You will know that the short-term discomfort, *is* short-term and that you'll benefit in the long term.

Your exposure therapy sessions

Preparing yourself

Before undertaking your treatment exercises, remind yourself why you are doing them. Go over your lists, and picture yourself doing all the activities you can't do now. Conjure up a positive but realistic version of yourself enjoying life without current restrictions. Then think something like: 'This is why I am about to confront my fears. I am providing myself with an opportunity to make my life better'.

Once you have dealt with general motivational issues, make a short list of specific preparation statements that you can use at the start of your exposure therapy sessions. Here are some examples:

- I'm feeling apprehensive, but that's normal at this stage
- When I start my exercise, I will feel uncomfortable, but I'll feel better the longer I stay with it
- I've got to do this to get better
- This will be uncomfortable in the short term, but there will be many long-term benefits
- I'm going to overcome this problem, I really am!
- Even if it feels bad, nothing terrible is going to happen; it just feels that way
- Take it easy: one step at a time.

Use a timetable

When undertaking a self-help programme, it is useful to pencil into a diary dates and times for practising planned tasks. Make sure that you set aside a reasonable amount of time – at least every other day – in which you can perform your exercises. You will probably need to set aside more time at the beginning of the programme. As you progress, exercises can be spaced out a little. Treat your exercises like hospital appointments: if you had made an appointment you would probably turn up on time, so, treat yourself with the same respect. Put a few minutes aside at the beginning of each session, and go over your reasons for undertaking the treatment plan. Then, read a few preparation statements, and keep them in your mind.

Finally, try to schedule your exposure sessions when you are not hassled or stessed. Attempting to enter a difficult situation when you are tired or upset is unlikely to be helpful; if your anxiety is already high, then it won't take much to make you feel panicky. However, if you undertake your exercises when you are feeling relatively calm and in control, the risk of panic is much reduced. Punctuating a relaxation exercise with preparation statements might be helpful.

Managing to cope

Coping statements are statements you use when you are actually undertaking your exposure exercises. Some people find it useful to prepare flash-cards that can be taken out and read at critical points. If you find your anxiety quite high at the beginning, then trying to remember coping statements might be too difficult. If this is the case, then write a statement down on a piece of card, and take it out at an appropriate moment. Don't just read it mechanically. Try to 'tune in' to the meaning of the statement. If you find that your heart rate is going up and your body is beginning to feel tense, take a deep breath, hold it for a few moments, and then breathe out slowly while thinking the word 'relax'. Every time you breathe out thereafter, think 'relax', or recite your coping statement.

Here are some examples of coping statements:

- I can cope with this
- My anxiety is up, but it has to come down
- I've got to accept my anxiety, it'll go down soon
- I knew it wasn't going to be easy, but I'm doing fine
- Relax: take a deep breath in, and breathe out slowly
- Things aren't really as bad as they seem
- Concentrate on what you're doing.

Afterwards: evaluation and praise

If you successfully accomplish your exercise, make sure you evaluate your efforts and praise yourself for your accomplishment. Look back over what you have done, and try to work out what helped you most. You may find that certain coping statements worked better than others. If so, use the most effective ones more in future. Recognize any gains, however small; progress is progress! If you are not used to evaluating and praising yourself, then maybe you should use prepared statements as before. Here are some more examples:

- I made some progress. It'll all add up in the end!
- I didn't think I'd cope, but I did!
- It wasn't as bad as I thought!
- I was anxious, but handled it all the same!
- I did it! Next time I'll do it better!
- Well done! That was a real achievement!

Challenging unhelpful thoughts

Thinking about things in a particular way can become a habit. We rarely stop and try to change the thoughts that routinely go through our heads. Our thoughts are so much a part of us, that we often accept them without hesitation as fact. If we treat our thoughts as facts, then they become capable of affecting how we behave. Challenging or questioning the validity of certain thoughts is central to 'cognitive therapy'.

Self-questioning

Unhelpful thoughts can be changed by challenging them. If a thought comes into your mind like: 'I've left my front door open', don't just accept it, stop and ask yourself a few questions:

- What is the evidence for this thought?
- Do I have any good reason to believe it?
- Am I not just confusing a thought with a fact?
- How many times have I gone back to check before, only to find the front door closed and locked?
- Given that I usually find my door closed and locked, is it very likely that it's open now?

- Even if the door is open, it doesn't mean someone will break in necessarily does it?

This kind of self-questioning can be very useful during response prevention. Remember, you've got more of a chance of resisting the urge to do something if you stop and think rationally about your situation than if you just react without thinking. You can apply this self-questioning to most habitual thoughts. For example, if you think that you are contaminated and must wash yourself, don't just accept it but stop, and ask yourself: What is the evidence? How do I know I've picked up a germ? Even if I have, how do I know it'll cause problems? Is it really likely? After questioning habitual thoughts, most people find that the thoughts are no longer as compelling. As always, practice is essential. It is unlikely that asking yourself a few questions on one or two occasions will have much impact on your thoughts and feelings. Challenging, and changing the way we think is a kind of mental discipline, and it's beneficial effects are usually closely related to practice and effort.

Help from members of your family

Before finishing this chapter, we should consider briefly the role of the family. If you live with your family, then it can be a very useful source of encouragement and support. However, encouragement and support can be distorted, and end up as reassurance. As already suggested seeking reassurance can be a subtle form of avoidance behaviour. So, you have to be careful.

If you do ask members of your family to help with your exposure tasks, make sure that your requests for help are not simply a way of avoiding the discomfort of taking full responsibility for your actions yourself. To avoid problems of this kind, get your family to agree on a particular phrase that they use in response to your requests for reassurance: for example, 'I don't think answering that question will be helpful' or 'I think it's best we don't talk about that'. Again, pre-prepared coping statements might be useful if you feel the urge to ask. For example:

- I'm asking questions here to reduce my discomfort, I don't need to do this
- Reassurance is not helpful to me in the long run, so I mustn't ask for it

- I can overcome my problems more successfully if I don't seek reassurance
- I must take full responsibility for my actions as soon as possible.

A word of warning though: *Don't* involve your family if your relationships are not good. Involving a partner, or parents, can be counterproductive if criticism or conflict is likely. Finally, in some families, particular individuals take on particular roles. These roles are usually associated with some kind of gain. As a result, the individual in question may have a vested interest in preserving his or her role. Usually these interests are not obvious, and are under the surface. For example, a mother may perceive herself as a caring person, and this role may be essential to her sense of self and purpose in life. As a result, when a member of the family becomes ill, she may have a vested interest in that person remaining ill. She may not be consciously thinking things like 'I hope the illness continues', but deep down this is what she wants and needs, and her behaviour may reflect this. Alternatively, a possessive husband might feel happier with his wife confined to the house because of a nervous problem, than if she recovered and became more independent. He may take on a protective role which, under the surface, shares more with the role of guard or warden.

If you suspect that members of your family have a vested interest in you remaining obsessional or anxious, then asking them for help is unlikely to be successful. Undertaking a self-help programme can be made virtually impossible, if your domestic environment contains a saboteur. Nevertheless you can use your newly-gained insight to your advantage and strengthen your resolve! What's more, you can always talk the problem over with your GP or a friend.

Summary

1. The preparation of helpful statements that can be recollected or read at times when anxiety is likely to influence thinking in a negative way can be very effective.
2. Helping statements can be used before (preparation), during (coping), and after (praise) undertaking a difficult exercise.
3. Preparation in a broader sense can take the form of scheduling exercises and considering motivational issues.
4. Challenging habitual and unhelpful thoughts can be employed as a means of resisting urges.

5. Family members can be a source of great support if relationships are good. It is useful to agree on standard responses to reassurance-seeking if reassurance is frequently employed to reduce anxiety.
6. Do not ask members of your family for help if you feel that they may be critical.

6

Exposure Therapy for Compulsive Washing and Cleaning

Compulsive washing and cleaning are usually due to a fear of contamination, a fear of contaminating others, yourself, or both. The following self-help programme will involve exposing yourself to places or things you consider to be 'dirty' or contaminated, resisting the urge to wash the contamination away, and allowing yourself less time to wash after resisting. In the final stages, washing might be omitted altogether. In Chapter 4, we learned about anxiety ladders, and used contamination fears as an example. We are going to use them again, but this time with you doing all the work.

The basic plan

1 First of all, write down a list of things and/or situations which make you feel uncomfortable and usually result in the urge to wash or clean. Be as specific as you can. (See Appendix III for charts etc for your own use.)
2 Give each of these situations an anxiety rating, using the following eight-point scale (see p. 54 for an example):

0	1	2	3	4	5	6	7	8
No anxiety		Slight anxiety		Moderate anxiety		Marked anxiety		Extreme anxiety

3 When you have rated all the situations, construct a five-step anxiety ladder (see p. 55), with the least upsetting situation at the bottom (step 1), and the most upsetting at the top (step 5).
4 Now consider the *least* upsetting situation, and ask yourself the following questions:

- How long could I reasonably maintain contact with the contaminant?
- How long could I reasonably wait without washing?
- What would be the minimum washing time I could cope with?

5 Construct a self-help plan so that every time you undertake exposure and response-prevention, you gradually:

- Increase your contact time with the contaminant
- Increase the interval between contamination and washing
- Reduce the time spent washing/cleaning

6 When you have exposed yourself to the situation to the extent that you no longer feel that washing is absolutely necessary, start work on the next item.

WORKED EXAMPLE

See Appendix III for blank charts for you to photocopy or copy out for your own use.

1 Things and situations which cause discomfort and usually result in the urge to wash:

> Touching a damp towel (at home)
> Touching a damp towel (at work)
> Sitting in certain chairs (at home)
> Sitting in certain chairs (at work)
> Shaking hands
> Faeces (e.g. dogs')
> Public baths
> Rain
> Handling uncooked vegetables
> Domestic pets
> Using the toilet (at home)
> Using the toilet (at work)
> Using a public toilet
> Touching library books
> Door handles (at work)
> Touching newspapers or magazines
> Eating in a restaurant
> Trying on clothes in a shop
> Touching the dustbin/emptying the dustbin
> Sitting near the wastepaper basket (at work)
> Walking past drains
> Walking past pet shops
> Going to the dentist

2 The things/situations rated using the eight-point anxiety scale:

Touching a damp towel (at home)	2
Touching a damp towel (at work)	7
Sitting in certain chairs (at home)	2
Sitting in certain chairs (at work)	4
Shaking hands	6
Faeces (e.g. dogs')	8
Public baths	8
Rain	3
Handling uncooked vegetables	5
Domestic pets	7
Using the toilet (at home)	4
Using the toilet (at work)	7
Using a public toilet	8
Touching library books	6
Door handles (at work)	6
Touching newspapers or magazines	5
Eating in a restaurant	7
Trying on clothes in a shop	7
Touching the dustbin	2
Emptying the dustbin	6
Sitting near the wastepaper basket (at work)	3
Walking past drains	7
Walking past pet shops	6
Going to the dentist	8

3 Construct a five-step anxiety ladder. Try to select situations or items which you can actually practise, and try to make each step go up by the same amount of anxiety. Although five steps are specified here, up to 10 would still be acceptable.

Step 5	Emptying the dustbin	6
Step 4	Touching newspapers or magazines	5
Step 3	Using the toilet (at home)	4
Step 2	Sitting near the wastepaper basket (at work)	3
Step 1	Touching the dustbin	2

4 Take Step 1, and specify times for initial contact, delay and washing/cleaning. For example:

Contact time:	1 minute
Delay:	3 minutes
Wash:	Not more than 5 minutes

5 Now construct an exposure and response-prevention plan. With every exposure, increase contact, extend delay and reduce wash times.

If you feel that you won't be able to cope with the rate of change shown below, then just stay with a particular combination of times until you feel ready to go on. For example:

Exposures	Time (min)		
	Contact	Delay	Wash
12	30	40	0
11	25	30	0
10	20	25	1
9	15	20	1
8	10	15	1
7	10	10	1
6	8	8	2
5	5	5	3
4	4	5	3
3	3	4	4
2	2	4	4
1	1	3	5

Notice that by the eleventh and twelfth exposures, response-prevention is total. It may seem odd to write a 30-minute delay into your programme, followed by no washing at all. The idea here is to continue extending delay times, irrespective of what actually happens. You might feel that a wash is necessary, even after delaying for 30 minutes. If that happens, then don't worry, try delaying for 40 minutes next time. The longer your delay time, the less likely you will feel the urge to wash. You might find that the urge to wash diminishes earlier than expected, for example after a 10-minute delay. If so, don't bother washing, just because it was permitted in your programme.

6 Having completed step one on the anxiety ladder (touching bin), it is now possible to move on to step two (here, sitting near waste paper basket). This will involve exactly the same principles. You might, for example, first try to spend five minutes sitting close to the basket. You could increase this, while delaying washing, and reducing wash time.

Additional detail

Below is a washing/cleaning diary (see Appendix III for copy to photocopy). You can fill it in before and after completing each exposure session. Where it says 'goals', write in the durations of time you intend to spend making contact with your contaminant, delaying, and washing. Tick appropriate boxes to show how long you were able to delay washing, and how long you spent washing. Also rate your discomfort/anxiety while resisting washing, and after washing; with the former, conduct your rating at the end of the delay period.

Washing/cleaning diary

Date: ....   Time: ....

Please specify item
(e.g. sink): ....

Goals: Contact time:.......... Delay:.......... Washing time:...........

Time spent delaying wash (Please tick)

Less than 1 minute ☐   About 1 minute   ☐
About 2 minutes   ☐   About 3 minutes   ☐
About 4 minutes   ☐   About 5 minutes   ☐
5–15 min ☐   15–30 ☐   30–45 ☐   45–1 hr ☐
1 hr–1 hr 30 min ☐   1 hr 30 min–2 hr ☐
2–3 hr ☐   3–4 ☐   4–5 ☐   5+ hr ☐
If more than 5 hr, please specify time ....

Discomfort/anxiety (when resisting)

0	1	2	3	4	5	6	7	8
Absent		Slight		Definite		Marked		Extreme

Time spent washing (Please tick)

Less than 1 minute ☐   About 1 minute   ☐
About 2 minutes   ☐   About 3 minutes   ☐
About 4 minutes   ☐   About 5 minutes   ☐
5–15 min ☐   15–30 ☐   30–45 ☐   45–1 hr ☐
1 hr–1 hr 30 min ☐   1 hr 30 min–2 hr ☐
2–3 hr ☐   3–4 ☐   4–5 ☐   5+ hr ☐
If more than 5 hr, please specify time ....

Discomfort/anxiety (After washing)

0	1	2	3	4	5	6	7	8
Absent		Slight		Definite		Marked		Extreme

You will find that initial resistance will be associated with relatively high levels of discomfort, and washing will be associated with considerable relief. However, as your exposure programme continues, you will find that resisting becomes easier, and washing is not associated with so much relief. You may even find that once you are up to delaying for an hour, you no longer even feel a strong urge to wash. *Complete* response prevention, when you feel up to it, should be written into your programme. This doesn't mean that you should never go near soap and water again! Rather it means that when your washing is no longer compulsive in nature, you can allow yourself to wash for a reasonable amount of time, like anybody else.

You may find that, as you feel less bothered by situations included on your anxiety ladder, other situations that are not included, become less frightening. This is a well-known phenomenon called 'generalization' (see p. 19) fortunately, coping also generalizes. If you become less frightened of several situations associated with contamination, it is likely that others will seem less frightening, even in the absence of direct exposure. So, don't worry too much about items that are difficult to include on your anxiety ladder (e.g. rain, hotel beds etc.). It is possible that your treatment gains will generalize, and that direct confrontation with unusual situations will not be necessary.

There may be some things which you regularly avoid contact with which need not be directly confronted at all. For example, if you avoid using parks because of dog faeces, then your exposure programme should involve walking in your local park (but obviously not touching the faeces which are likely to be contaminated). There is no need to learn to tolerate touching things that the average person does not come into contact with during the course of everyday life.

Lastly, don't trick yourself. During exposure sessions, some people with obsessive–compulsive disorder cope with their anxiety by defining 'acceptable' areas, or performing covert rituals – for example, only touching a small part of a toilet seat designated 'germ free'; or, while touching the toilet seat, thinking 'magic' words, to ward off infection. These are simply further examples of avoidance, and should be stopped immediately.

Skin care

Excessive contact with water can lead to a depletion of natural oils, causing skin to become dry and scaly. Excessive washing and use of detergents (even hand soap) can lead to the development of an irritant dermatitis in which the skin becomes inflamed. Continual irritation might even result in eczema. Older people are more vulnerable to these problems than younger people because their skin is already considerably dryer.

Many people with obsessional problems wash so frequently that they develop skin conditions like those described above. These can be very painful, especially if the skin cracks. In addition, skin conditions can be embarrassing. Many obsessional washers develop sore hands; these are relatively exposed and easily noticed by relatives or acquaintances. A question like 'What have you done to your hands?' can be very distressing, even if asked with the best intentions. When you are making great efforts to hide your obsessional problem, visible symptoms, such as soreness, can be most unwelcome.

Redness, soreness, itching and cracked skin may be reduced by using any fragrance-free moisturizer. The Simple, or Neutragena ranges are examples which can be bought at your local chemist. Many people with sore skin use E-45 cream, however, which is probably unwise: E-45 contains lanolin, which is a fat-like substance derived from the wool of sheep. Animal products like this may sensitize the skin further, leading to the development of an allergy. If you can't find Simple or Neutragena products, any moisturizer will do, providing it is not scented and does not contain lanolin.

If you moisturize your hands regularly this may reduce your discomfort, and relieve some of your more obvious symptoms; however, if your skin problems persist, you should go and see your GP for further advice. He or she may need to refer you to a dermatologist – a doctor who specializes in skin care.

Compulsive washing is an attempt to reduce the chances of getting an infection. When taken to an extreme, the behaviour becomes self-defeating. Washing to the point where your skin becomes dry and cracked is likely to *increase* the chances of infection, rather than reduce it. Remember this fact when attempting to change your washing behaviour. It may help you to reduce the time you spend washing.

Summary

1. Compulsive washing can be treated using exposure sessions, self-imposed delay, and response-prevention.
2. Do not designate 'germ free' areas during exposure sessions.
3. Do not undertake any covert or mental rituals to reduce anxiety.

7

Exposure Therapy and Other Techniques for Compulsive Checking

Compulsive checking is usually due to an excessive sense of responsibility. The individual fears that through negligence, something untoward might happen, causing harm to others and incurring blame.

The basic plan for exposure and response-prevention in treating compulsive checking is much the same as that described for the treatment of compulsive washing and cleaning (Chapter 6). If you skipped that chapter, don't worry, all the main points will be repeated here; however, a good understanding of Chapters 2, 3 and 4 is essential.

The basic plan

1 Write down a list of the things that you check excessively. Be as specific as you can (see Appendix III for charts etc. for your use).
2 Give each of these items an anxiety rating, using the following eight-point anxiety scale. Imagine how anxious you would feel if you were unable to check. Some 'checkers' are unhappy with the term 'anxiety' and prefer to use 'discomfort' instead. If this is the case for you, just treat the anxiety scale as a general discomfort scale. Anxiety and discomfort both respond to exposure and response-prevention.

0	1	2	3	4	5	6	7	8
No anxiety/ discomfort		Slight anxiety/ discomfort		Moderate anxiety/ discomfort		Marked anxiety/ discomfort		Extreme anxiety/ discomfort

3 When you have rated all the items you check excessively, construct a five-step anxiety ladder, with the least upsetting at the bottom (Step 1), and the most upsetting at the top (Step 5).
4 Consider the least upsetting first. Now ask yourself the following:

- At first, what would be the minimum number of checks acceptable?
- If I got the urge to go back and check, how long would it be reasonable for me to resist?
- On my return, what minimum number of checks should I allow myself?

5 Construct a self-help plan so that every time you undertake exposure and response-prevention, you gradually:

- Reduce the number of initial checks
- Increase the interval between initial checks and final checks
- Reduce the number of final checks

6 As you increase your delay time, you will find that your urge to check diminishes. Try to cope with *not* going back to check as soon as you can. When you are able to check only once, and your resistance to returning is accompanied by minimal discomfort, repeat the above procedure on the next item up on your anxiety ladder.

WORKED EXAMPLE

See Appendix III for blank charts for you to photocopy or copy out for your own use.

1   Things that are checked excessively:

Windows (when leaving the house)
Cooker (after use)
Iron (after use)
Front door (when leaving the house)
Back door (irrespective of leaving)
Computer (at work)
Letters (re-opening to see if correspondence is inside)
Coffee machine (after use)
Car door (when leaving)
Retracing steps (to see if something has been dropped)
Fridge (after use)
Bathroom taps (after use)
Kitchen taps (irrespective of use)
Kitchen light switch (irrespective of use)
Bathroom light switch (after use)
Bedroom light switch (after use)

2 The anxiety/discomfort experienced by you when not able to check these items rated using the eight-point scale:

Windows (when leaving the house)	2
Cooker (after use)	7
Iron (after use)	8
Front door (when leaving the house)	8
Back door (irrespective of leaving)	7
Computer (at work)	5
Letters (re-opening to see if correspondence is inside)	6
Coffee machine (after use)	3
Car door (when leaving)	4
Retracing steps (to see if something has been dropped)	7
Fridge (after use)	5
Bathroom taps (after use)	6
Kitchen taps (irrespective of use)	6
Kitchen light switch (irrespective of use)	3
Bathroom light switch (after use)	2
Bedroom light switch (after use)	2

3 Construct a five-step anxiety ladder. Try to select situations or items which you can practise, and try to make each step go up by the same amount of anxiety. Although five steps are specified here, up to 10 would still be acceptable.

Step 5	Kitchen taps (irrespective of use)	6
Step 4	Fridge (after use)	5
Step 3	Car door (when leaving)	4
Step 2	Coffee machine (after use)	3
Step 1	Bedroom light switch (after use)	2

4 Take Step 1, and specify initial number of checks, delay time, and final number of checks. You might find it useful to make a distinction between minor checks and major checks. A minor check is a very swiftly accomplished check (for example a quick look around the edge of a door to make sure that it is closed, or shaking the door handle), whereas a major check is a return journey after leaving.

For example:

	Minor	Major
Initial Number of Checks:	6	3
Delay:	3 min	
Final Checks:	3	1

5 Now construct an exposure and response-prevention plan. With every exposure, reduce the initial number of checks, increase the delay and reduce final number of checks.

If you feel that you won't be able to cope with the rate of change shown below, then just stay with a particular combination until you feel ready to move on.

For example:

Exposures	Initial Minor	Major	Delay	Final Minor	Major
10	1	0	45	0	0
9	1	0	30	0	0
8	1	0	20	1	1
7	1	0	15	1	1
6	2	1	10	1	1
5	3	1	10	2	1
4	4	2	8	2	1
3	4	2	5	2	1
2	5	3	4	3	1
1	6	3	3	3	1

Notice that by the ninth exposure, final checks have been omitted completely. Obviously, it is impossible to do a final minor check in the absence of a major check. Similarly, it is impossible to do a final major in the absence of at least one minor check. It might seem odd to write a 30- or 45-minute delay, into your programme, followed by no checks (e.g. ninth and tenth exposures). This is of course, total response-prevention, rather than self-imposed delay. The idea here is to continue extending delay times, irrespective of what actually happens. You might feel that one last check is necessary, even after delaying for 30 minutes. If that happens, then don't worry, try delaying for 45 minutes next time. The longer your delay time, the less likely you will feel the urge to return to check. You might find that the urge to check diminishes earlier than expected, for example after a 10-minute delay. If so, don't bother going back, even if you planned to do so in your programme.

6 Having completed step one on the anxiety ladder (e.g. bedroom light switch), it is now possible to move on to step two (coffee machine). This will involve exactly the same principles.

Additional details

Below is a checking diary (see Appendix III for copy to photocopy). You can fill it in before and after completing each session. Where it says 'goals', write in the initial checks, delay time, and number of final checks. Tick appropriate boxes to show how long you spent checking initially, and finally (where appropriate). Also rate your

Checking Diary 1

Date: ....   Time: ....

Please specify item
(e.g. door): ....

Goals:	Initial	Check	Delay time	Final	Check
	Minor	*Major*	*Minutes*	*Minor*	*Major*
Number	_____	_____	_____	_____	_____

Time spent checking initially (Please tick)

Less than 1 minute   ☐   About 1 minute   ☐
About 2 minutes   ☐   About 3 minutes   ☐
About 4 minutes   ☐   About 5 minutes   ☐
5–15 min ☐   15–30 ☐   30–45 ☐   45–1 hr ☐
1 hr–1 hr 30 min ☐   1 hr 30 min–2 hr ☐
2–3 hr ☐   3–4 ☐   4–5 ☐   5+ hr ☐
If more than 5 hr, please specify time ....

Discomfort/Anxiety (when resisting)

0	1	2	3	4	5	6	7	8
Absent		Slight		Definite		Marked		Extreme

Time spent checking finally (Please tick)

Less than 1 minute   ☐   About 1 minute   ☐
About 2 minutes   ☐   About 3 minutes   ☐
About 4 minutes   ☐   About 5 minutes   ☐
5–15 min ☐   15–30 ☐   30–45 ☐   45–1 hr ☐
1 hr–1 hr 30 min ☐   1 hr 30 min–2 hr ☐
2–3 hr ☐   3–4 ☐   4–5 ☐   5+ hr ☐
If more than 5 hr, please specify time ....

Discomfort/Anxiety (after final check)

0	1	2	3	4	5	6	7	8
Absent		Slight		Definite		Marked		Extreme

Checking Diary 2

Date: ....   Time: ....

Please specify item
(e.g. door): ....

Goals:	Initial *Minor*	Check *Major*	Delay time *Minutes*	Final *Minor*	Check *Major*
Number	_____	_____	_____	_____	_____

Number of actual checks

Initial

	Minor	Major			Minor	Major
One	☐	☐	Ten to	15	☐	☐
Two	☐	☐	15 to	20	☐	☐
Three	☐	☐	20 to	25	☐	☐
Four	☐	☐	30 to	40	☐	☐
Five	☐	☐	40 to	50	☐	☐
Six	☐	☐	50 to	75	☐	☐
Seven	☐	☐	75 to	100	☐	☐
Eight	☐	☐	More than 100		☐	☐
Nine	☐	☐	More than 200		☐	☐
Ten	☐	☐	More than 300		☐	☐

Discomfort/Anxiety (when resisting)

0	1	2	3	4	5	6	7	8
Absent		Slight		Definite		Marked		Extreme

Number of actual checks

Final

	Minor	Major			Minor	Major
One	☐	☐	Ten to	15	☐	☐
Two	☐	☐	15 to	20	☐	☐
Four	☐	☐	30 to	40	☐	☐
Five	☐	☐	40 to	50	☐	☐
Six	☐	☐	50 to	75	☐	☐
Seven	☐	☐	75 to	100	☐	☐
Eight	☐	☐	More than 100		☐	☐
Nine	☐	☐	More than 200		☐	☐
Ten	☐	☐	More than 300		☐	☐

Discomfort/Anxiety (after final check)

0	1	2	3	4	5	6	7	8
Absent		Slight		Definite		Marked		Extreme

---

discomfort while resisting, and after your final check. With the former, conduct your rating at the end of the delay period.

A second checking diary is also included. This is exactly the same as the first, except instead of including boxes for recording the time you spend checking, it includes boxes that can be ticked to record the number of checks that you actually perform. Some people prefer to monitor their checking behaviour in this way. There are no advantages or disadvantages, it is simply a matter of preferences. Discomfort while resisting remains the best measure of change.

Making progress

Initially, resistance will be associated with relatively high levels of discomfort, and checking will bring about considerable relief. However, you will find that as your exposure programme continues, resisting becomes easier, and your final checks are not associated with so much relief. You may even find that once you are up to delaying for 30 minutes or an hour, you no longer feel a strong urge to check at all. *Complete* response prevention should be written into your programme when you feel up to it. This does not mean that you should never check anything again! Rather, that when your checking is no longer compulsive in nature, you can allow yourself to check things as reasonably as anybody else.

You may find that, as you feel less bothered by situations included on your anxiety ladder, other situations that are not included become less worrying. This is a well-known phenomenon called generalization (see p. 19). Fortunately, coping also generalizes. If you worry less about several situations associated with checking, it is likely that others will seem less worrying, even in the absence of direct exposure. So, do not concern yourself too much about items which are difficult to include on your anxiety ladder (e.g. checking behaviours which occur at work). It is possible that your treatment gains will generalize, and that direct confrontation with inconvenient situations will not be necessary.

If you suffer a marked increase in anxiety when checking, this does not mean that exposure therapy and response-prevention are not applicable to you; the programme outlined above is still relevant. Some checkers complain that the more they check, the more anxious or uncomfortable they feel. This might be due to the fact that if you do the same thing, over and over again, it has the effect of making your activity less distinct. A behaviour that is not distinctive, is less easily remembered, and confusion about whether or not an action was performed correctly, can lead to doubt. Such doubts can increase discomfort and anxiety. If this is your experience, then doubt-reduction procedures may be helpful. These will be considered shortly.

If you find that repeated checking makes you feel worse, rather than better, then this insight might be used therapeutically. You could say to yourself: 'I've checked once, and that is enough. If I continue to check it'll just make me feel worse. If I stop now, this will be the most discomfort I have to deal with. This level of discomfort will reduce to tolerable levels, in a shorter time, if I refrain from checking again.'

Other supplementary techniques

Imagined exposure

Research has shown that 'checkers' respond better to behavioural therapy when they have been exposed to the situations which they fear the most – in imagination only. Compulsive checkers report feeling quite anxious when *thinking* through a feared situation, but with continued exposure, they can get used to it. As usual, anxiety goes up, stays there for a while, and then comes down again. Repeated practice imagining the situation can reduce anxiety. As anxiety levels get lower, the urge to check is greatly reduced. This is because the upsetting thoughts and images are no longer as distressing as they were previous to exposure.

In a consultation, the patient might lie down, relax, and begin to describe a situation that s/he fears as though it were actually happening. The patient would be instructed to try to imagine the scene in detail. Occasionally, the therapist might stop the patient and say something like 'What's happening now?' or 'Hold that image for a few moments longer'. Particularly upsetting images are held in the mind until the anxiety lessens. In the absence of a therapist, you must learn to detect the most upsetting images, and hold them in your mind's eye.

You can try making up your own scenarios. You may be able to do this without any trouble. On the other hand, you might find writing down a detailed account of one of your scenarios, and making a cassette tape recording helpful. You can then play the recording to yourself, while you imagine what is being described. Keep playing the tape of your imagined scenario until your anxiety level goes down.

Here is an example of an imagined catastrophic 'scenario':

> I'm leaving the house. It's a cold morning, and I don't check the door properly. I am the last to leave. My mother and father have already gone out, and I am entirely responsible for anything that might happen. A stranger is walking down my road. He is walking very slowly, and looking at each house as he passes. There is nobody else around. When he gets to my house he stops, and notices that the door is not closed. He opens the front gate, and walks down the path. In a few moments, he is in the house. He immediately runs up the stairs, and goes into my mother and father's bedroom. He opens the drawers of the dressing table, and rummages around, occasionally throwing things on to the floor. He finds my mother's jewellery box, and opens it. He smiles as he sees her rings and two bracelets. One of the rings has special sentimental value to my mother. She once said it was irreplacable. Lifting them out of the box, the burglar places them into his pocket, and runs down the stairs. He peeps out, nobody is coming. He then slips out of the house, and runs off.
>
> I am now returning from work, late. I get out of the car, and notice a police car is parked outside my house. When I get inside, I walk into the lounge. My mother is sitting down, with my father next to her, holding her hand. She has been crying. A policeman is standing by the table. My mother looks up and says: 'We've been robbed. All my jewellery has been stolen'. I sit down, and feel sick with guilt. The policeman says 'The lock wasn't forced. Is it possible you left it open this morning? I say 'Yes, I suppose it is possible.' I begin to feel very anxious and notice that my mother and father are looking at me with stern expressions on their faces.

Imagined exposure is an optional technique. You don't have to do it if you don't want to. As suggested earlier, some people, but not all, find it helpful. You might like to try it, just to see if it does help. If not, then just carry on with your exposure and response-prevention programme.

Doubt-reduction procedures
Checking is very closely associated with the experience of doubt.

The compulsive checker often feels compelled to check, because he or she doubts whether a particular action has been accomplished. If we can reduce the level of doubt an individual experiences, this might be accompanied by a reduction in the urge to check.

Some kind of memory problem might be an important contributory factor to feelings of doubt. It may be that checkers doubt whether something has been properly accomplished, because they can't remember it very well. On the other hand, it may be that they are pretty sure that they did whatever it was, but have no confidence in their memory; in other words, the 'recollection' just doesn't provide enough evidence to stop them from doubting. So, doubt might occur because of a deficient memory, or a lack of confidence in memory.

Most checking behaviours are not distinctive. They are all quite similar, and therefore, easy to forget. If you make a particular 'check' very distinctive, then it might be easier to remember, and reduce your doubting. So, how can we make our checking more noticeable, and easier to recall. Here are a few ideas.

Memory technique (1)

Find some thin, coloured cardboard (you can buy this in any stationers; section divides for folders would do) and cut out four different shapes in three sizes: large, medium, and small. The exact sizes do not matter, although they should be able to fit into a shirt, jacket or skirt pocket. A rough guide would be to make each group of shapes about 8 cm (large), 6 cm (medium) and 4cm (small) high (see Table 2). Keep the sets separate, and note the following instructions.

Table 2: Set of distinctive shapes for use as part of memory technique (1).

☆	L	M	S	(Blue)
□	L	M	S	(Green)
△	L	M	S	(Red)
○	L	M	S	(Yellow)

Key: L=large; M=medium; S=small

---

1 When you are about to do something which usually leads to checking, take one of the large shapes, and look at it for a few moments. Associate your activity with the shape and its colour. For example, when leaving the house, close the door, take out the large triangle, and make an association between the closed door and the large triangle.

2 When you have finished your activity, and feel the urge to check, remind yourself that the activity was successfully completed by imagining the particular shape associated with the activity and its colour.

3 Use a different large shape every time you undertake the activity. When you have worked through all the colours of a particular size, start using shapes the next size down. So, after using the large star, triangle, square, and circle, go on to the medium-sized shapes. After the medium-sized shapes, work through the small shapes.

4 When you have finished using the smallest shapes, undertake your activity without using the shapes, but imagining them instead. For instance, you might close the door and think of a red triangle.

A different coloured shape is employed every time, so that each final check is made more distinctive, or unique. As suggested earlier, distinctive things are easier to remember. The shapes gradually become smaller as part of a procedure called fading. Using coloured pieces of card can be a little inconvenient, so once they have done their job, it is necessary to fade them out. Some people find that after fading them out, they no longer need to imagine shapes; having got used to not checking, they feel that they don't need to any more. Others find that imagining distinctive shapes continues to be helpful. If you find the fade described above a little too fast, make more shapes with a larger range of sizes – for example, sets of five (extra large, large, medium, small, and very small) (see Table 3).

A hint: some people find that when starting this technique, imagining the shapes to alleviate doubt isn't enough. They have found it useful to look at the shape again, and remind themselves that the last time they saw it was, for example, by the closed door. After doing this a few times, imagining the shape is usually sufficient to alleviate doubt on its own.

Table 3: Enlarged set of distinctive shapes for use as part of memory technique (1).

☆	XL	L	M	S	VS	(Blue)
▢	XL	L	M	S	VS	(Green)
△	XL	L	M	S	VS	(Red)
◯	XL	L	M	S	VS	(Yellow)
▢	XL	L	M	S	VS	(Orange)

Key: XL = extra large; L = large; M = medium; S = small; VS = very small.

As usual, if this technique helps you, then use it, if it doesn't, then just continue with your basic exposure and response-prevention plan. A few patients have found it useful as a temporary measure: they started off using the shapes at the beginning of their programmes until they felt confident. Once they became comfortable with their programme, then response prevention was undertaken without the use of coloured figures. As such, it can be employed as a 'bridging manoeuvre' or 'exposure aid'.

Memory technique 2

If you make your final check distinctive, you are less likely to doubt whether you did it or not. One very simple way of making a check distinctive is to associate it with a unique image or mental picture. The more bizarre the image is, the more likely you are to remember it. For example, when turning off the gas cooker, you might imagine a miniature version of Luciano Pavarotti sitting on the back burner singing 'No need to check' to the tune of *Nessun dorma*! Again, this is a rather unconventional technique, which might, or might not, be helpful. It is less systematic than the shape technique, and does not have the advantage of 'built in' fading, although one might simply imagine smaller and smaller images. Nevertheless, some commentators have suggest that unique imagery can be employed successfully to alleviate doubts and as such, it might be worth trying.

Techniques for 'retracers'

It was suggested earlier that some people with obsessive–compulsive disorder retrace their steps to see if they have been the cause of an accident. The construction of an exposure and response-prevention hierarchy for this kind of checking isn't obvious, so here are some hints. The checking behaviour occurs in order to reduce anxiety stemming from thoughts about harming others, and subsequent blame. Sensitivity to responsibility and a low tolerance of guilt are also associated features.

Exposure to upsetting thoughts about harming others can be achieved by using the imagined-exposure technique described earlier. You can write a series of scenarios, of increasing levels of unpleasantness, and imagine them for longer and longer periods of time. You can also expose yourself to related upsetting thoughts by using habituation training (Chapter 9). Self-imposed delay and response-prevention can be employed in a similar way as described above. For example, if you feel compelled to go back and check, then stop and resist. Wait for as long as you can before allowing yourself to check. Every time you get the urge to retrace your steps, see if you can wait a little longer.

A number of obsessive–compulsive disorder patients say that after checking the site of an imagined accident, they doubt the accuracy of their memory. They also complain that they are not confident that their checking was sufficient. Doubt might be reduced by using one of the memory techniques described above. For example, when you return to the scene of the imagined accident, take out a memory card, and say something to yourself like 'I have checked sufficiently. There are no signs of an accident. I do not need to come back again.' After leaving, when you get the urge to check, look at your memory card, and use it to remind yourself that you have checked sufficiently, that there were no signs of an accident, and that you don't need to go back. Once you have reduced your doubt, resistance should be easier. Try to stop going back completely as soon as possible. By using a combination of techniques (imagined exposure, habituation training, self-imposed delay, a doubt-reduction procedure, and response-prevention) you should be able to overcome this very difficult problem.

Summary

1. Obsessional checking can be treated by exposure, self-imposed

delay, and response-prevention.

2. An exposure and response-prevention programme may be supplemented by several other techniques. Exposing yourself to imagined (catastrophic) outcomes, may, over time, reduce your initial levels of anxiety. Further, doubt may be alleviated by increasing the uniqueness of checks by associating them with distinctive symbols or distinctive images.

3. Memory techniques can be used in conjunction with your exposure and response-prevention programme. Alternatively, they can be used to help reduce doubt as you get started.

8

Self-help for Slowness, Symmetry and Hoarding

Although washing and checking are the most common obsessional behaviours there are several others which deserve some mention, even though they are comparatively rare. These are primary obsessional slowness, the need for symmetry, and hoarding. Each, in its own way, reflects a personality trait described as part of the obsessional personality; it may be the case that these kinds of obsession overlap with obsessive–compulsive personality disorder considerably.

Primary obsessional slowness

Primary obsessional slowness was recognized diagnostically only relatively recently. Certain patients complained that simple every-day tasks were taking a long time to complete. This wasn't because they were stopping to check things, it was simply because they were slow. This 'slowness' was particularly apparent during the comple-tion of everyday tasks, such as getting ready in the morning, washing, or shaving. Some of the patients were taking up to 30 minutes to clean their teeth. When asked why they were taking so long, many of the patients found it difficult to explain why; however, the root of the problem appears to be a desire to do things in a meticulous or 'correct' way, i.e. to a very high standard.

Treatment usually starts with a therapist 'modelling' (i.e. demon-strating) a problem behaviour at an appropriate speed. The patient then undertakes that behaviour, while the therapist urges him or her on at regular intervals. Usually, a goal time is set at the beginning of each session, and the patient tries to accomplish his or her task within the set limit.

If you are accustomed to doing things slowly, then regular prompts and time limits might lead to discomfort associated with being 'hassled' or rushed. Surprisingly, few patients respond badly to this approach; the worse that happens is a slight increase in irritability and a loss of concentration.

Treatment

Treatment for primary obsessional slowness may be rather difficult in the absence of a therapist to model and prompt. Nevertheless, it is still possible to help yourself with regard to setting time limits. Here are some basic instructions.

1. Write down a list of tasks which usually take you a long time.
2. Note down approximately how long each one takes to complete. Order them, so that the slowest are at the top of the page, and the quickest at the bottom.
3. Select one of your tasks, from near the bottom of your list, and time how long it takes you to complete it from start to finish. Now set a goal time that you think would be more reasonable.
4. Repeat the task, as often as usual, but reducing the time you allow yourself by a minute each session. Stop when you have reached your goal time. Practise at this speed until you are comfortable with it, then apply the same principles to another task further up on your list.

Your treatment plan might look something like this (see Appendix III for your copy):

Washing teeth

Current time taken: 10 minutes

Goal time:	4 minutes
	Time allowed
Session 7	4 minutes
Session 6	5 minutes
Session 5	6 minutes
Session 4	7 minutes
Session 3	8 minutes
Session 2	9 minutes
Session 1	10 minutes

Although you might not have a therapist to prompt you, there are other ways of providing yourself with prompts. Obviously, a member of your family could be asked. If you find this unacceptable, then you can employ a number of mechanical aids. Many new watches and personal organizers have multiple alarm settings. You could get set two alarms in each session. One to tell you that you are half-way through, and a second to tell you that it's time to stop. This sometimes helps to sustain an appropriate pace, especially during long sessions early on in treatment.

Symmetry and order

Sometimes people develop obsessions to do with order and symmetry. For example, things must be taken out of a draw in a certain order; or, things must be lined up in a particular way. Usually, when people with this kind of obsession are interrupted mid-ritual, they feel that they have to go back to the beginning and start again.

As with obsessional slowness, people who have obsessions to do with order do not necessarily know why; however, it is likely that a kind of superstitious thinking underlies the problem. The individual might get a thought like: 'If I don't keep my books in alphabetical order, my father will be involved in an accident'. The individual may acknowledge that thinking like this is completely irrational, but at the back of his or her mind, he or she might be thinking: 'What if it were to happen? What if my father did die in an accident? I would feel dreadful. I would blame myself'. This kind of thinking results in increased anxiety, which is reduced by putting the books in order. The individual might then think: 'If something happens now, I won't feel that I was negligent'. Of course, nothing happens, so the superstitious behaviour appears to be successful. Because the likelihood of a serious accident is so low, any superstitious behaviour designed to ward off such occurrences will appear to work. New learning only occurs when the behaviour isn't performed. The individual then has the opportunity to learn that special order and symmetry are serving no useful function.

Symmetry and order compulsion might be comparable to checking. Things have to be done in a certain way to avoid harm to self or others. Whereas there is a logical link between checking the gas fire several times and worry about the house burning down, there is no obvious link between worries about accidents, and ordering things. Although worrying about future accidents is used in our example, obsessional thoughts that prompt order rituals can be about anything that makes the individual anxious. Further, symmetry rituals can occur in the absence of obsessional thoughts altogether. The individual might just feel uncomfortable about a lack of order, and relieve the tension by lining things up, or by executing some kind of 'balancing' activity.

Treatment

Compulsive ordering can be treated in exactly the same way as checking. The individual exposes him or herself to situations usually associated with an 'order' ritual, and then resists the urge. Anxiety goes up, and then after a while, comes down. Repetition will eventually result in reduced anxiety and new learning.

Here is an example of an exposure and response-prevention plan for somebody who, when scratching his face on one side, feels that he then has to scratch his face on the other side too, in the exact opposite place.

Exposure	Scratch 1	Delay	Scratch 2
8	Scratch	1 hour	
7	Scratch 1	30 minutes	–
6	Scratch 1	20 minutes	–
5	Scratch 1	15 minutes	Scratch 2
4	Scratch 1	10 minutes	Scratch 2
3	Scratch 1	8 minutes	Scratch 2
2	Scratch 1	4 minutes	Scratch 2
1	Scratch 1	1 minute	Scratch 2

Notice that on the sixth exposure session, the individual in question planned to resist scratching a second time altogether.

Progress could be recorded using the following type of form:

Date: ....   Time: ....

Please specify item: e.g. Scratching opposite side of face, after scratching an itch.

Goals: Delay time:

Discomfort scale (e.g when resisting scratching):

0	1	2	3	4	5	6	7	8
Absent		Slight		Definite		Marked		Extreme

Discomfort scale (e.g. after second scratch):

0	1	2	3	4	5	6	7	8
Absent		Slight		Definite		Marked		Extreme

Anxiety/discomfort ratings will be high at first. The second scratch will also be associated with much relief; however, as the delay times increase, it will become easier to resist the second scratch.

Obsessional counting

Another aspect of order rituals is obsessional counting. For example, an obsessional checker may need to rattle a door handle in multiples of 4, until satisfied that the door is closed. A counting sequence might go something like this: 1,2,3,4 . . . 5,6,7,8 . . . 9,10,11,12. These habits are quite difficult to break; however, some people find it easier to conquer counting rituals if they jumble up their numbers. Checking is, at first, allowed but only if counting goes something like this: 4,2,3,1, . . . 7,2,9,1 . . . 4,11,9,2. Eventually, attempts are made to stop counting completely.

Hoarding

A hoarding obsession can take many forms. For example, it can involve storing more food than can possibly be eaten, or collecting something completely useless like bits of waste paper. At worst, an individual might fill his or her home with something completely useless, finding it impossible to throw the collected items away. Again, a behavioural treatment will involve resisting collection, and waiting for discomfort to diminish. Gradually increasing the delay time will result in a decrease in the urge to collect. This can also be complemented by a programme of throwing things away in stages. So, for sombody who hoards old newspapers, throwing away the daily paper might be a useful way of starting. Once the individual is comfortable with throwing away the daily paper, each 'throw away' can be accompanied by one old copy. This can then be stepped up, so that each daily 'throw away' is accompanied by two old papers, then three, and so on.

Summary

1. Primary obsessional slowness, the need for symmetry, and hoarding, are all more unusual examples of obsessive–compulsive disorder.
2. It is possible that these are more closely related to obsessive–compulsive personality disorder; however, there is insufficient evidence to support a strong link at this stage.

3. Irrespective of their diagnostic status, all are to some degree responsive to behavioural treatments.
4. Modifications of the basic exposure and response prevention plan are recommended.

9

Dealing with Upsetting Thoughts and Excessive Worry

Some people complain of obsessions, in the absence of compulsions. Although these 'pure obsessions' do exist alone, more often than not they are associated with anxiety-reducing rituals which are performed mentally.

There is also a kind of intrusive thought called 'morbid preoccupation'. These are slightly different from obsessions, and are closer to what might be described as excessive worry. Nevertheless, morbid preoccupations are similar to obsessions, in that both are experienced as unpleasant, and difficult to control, and both can be alleviated by certain techniques.

Exposure therapy and habituation

Thoughts are, of course, unpredictable; they can also be 'fleeting', and difficult to hold in your mind – especially if they make you anxious. Theoretically, repeated exposure to an upsetting thought should result in decreased anxiety. To expose yourself to your obsessional thought, you have first to capture it. You must be in a position to control the thought, and expose yourself to it whenever it is convenient. In this way, you can learn to tolerate the thought for an amount of time, sufficient to allow your anxiety to habituate.

There are several strategies which can allow you to do this. The first is simply to practice forming the upsetting thought, and then holding it in your mind; however, as suggested above, not everybody can do this, because thoughts can be very 'slippery'. A second strategy is to write your thought down on a piece of paper, and to keep on looking at it. A variation of this is simply to write, and re-write the thought for a set period of time. Although this technique can be effective, it has the problem of not being very realistic. The experiences of writing a thought down, and of 'hearing' it inside your head are quite different. Ideally, your exposure programme should be as realistic as possible. With the third technique, you are asked to speak your thought, or thoughts, while recording them onto a 'loop tape'. (A loop tape simply goes round and round, repeating whatever has been recorded. You can get them at most good audio shops.) By using a personal stereo (e.g. a Walkman), an individual can walk around, exposing him or herself to an obsessional thought, in a controlled and predictable way. The incessant repetition of the upsetting thought should also discourage the listener from performing neutralizing, anxiety-reducing rituals.

Loop-tape technique

1 First of all, write a list of your upsetting thoughts. Rate them for the amount of discomfort or anxiety associated with each using the following eight-point scale.

0	1	2	3	4	5	6	7	8
No anxiety		Slight anxiety		Moderate anxiety		Marked anxiety		Extreme anxiety

Then, place your thoughts on a five-step anxiety ladder, with the least upsetting thought at the bottom (step 1), and the most upsetting thought at the top (step 5). If you have only one obsessional thought, then clearly this is not necessary.

2 Record your least upsetting thought on a 'loop tape'. Usually, the loop tape will repeat your thought every 30 seconds.

3 Play the tape for about 15 minutes, and rate discomfort or anxiety at regular intervals. About once every three minutes would be fine.

Set your ratings out like this:

Minutes	Ratings
3	——
6	——
9	——
12	——
15	——

Listen to the tape very carefully. When your obsessional thought occurs, do not distract yourself, and don't undertake any mental rituals to make things right, or to cancel the obsessional thought's effect.

4 Practise listening to your thought at least twice a day, for one hour. Do this until your anxiety or discomfort is down by about

half compared to initial levels. Ratings do not have to be every three minutes. You might try every five minutes at first, then every 10 minutes.

Although the ratings are there to monitor your emotional response to the thoughts, the fact that you have to rate them does make you listen more carefully. This is a good thing, because otherwise you might get used to the tape and just 'switch off'. For the technique to be effective, you have to 'engage' in the task.

5 Once you are relatively comfortable with your least upsetting obsessional thought, then exchange it for the next one up on your anxiety ladder. Carry on doing this until you experience anxiety reduction with all your obsessional thoughts.

Additional details

It is usually the case that after exposure has been successfully accomplished on two or three thoughts, the effect generalizes. The remaining upsetting thoughts begin to lose their potency, reducing the necessity for formal exposure sessions.

Certain upsetting thoughts are associated with particular situations. For example, an obsessional thought like 'I'm going to stab someone' might only occur in the supermarket. If so, you can consolidate your therapeutic gains by undertaking further exposure sessions in the feared situation itself. In our present example, this would involve wearing your personal stereo and listening to your thought in the supermarket.

If this seems frightening to you, then as before, do it in stages. Go into the supermarket and listen to your thought once. Then try listening to it for one minute. Slowly work up to tolerating your thought for the full duration of your shopping trip. Remember, on no account distract or undertake covert rituals whilst doing this exercise. This will only impair the efficiency of this technique.

Thought management techniques

Thought-stopping

Thought-stopping is a technique which is usually undertaken with a therapist present. The patient tries to summon up the obsessional thought and indicates its presence by lifting a finger. At this point, the therapist shouts 'Stop!'. The shout might also be accompanied by a loud noise (e.g. banging a ruler or clapping). This noisy interruption sometimes results in the mind clearing.

After this has been practised, the patient repeats the procedure without assistance. As the obsessional thought begins to form, he or she shouts 'Stop!', and as before, the effect is one of mind clearance. The process is then repeated, and on every repetition the volume of the 'Stop!' is reduced slightly. Eventually, the 'Stop!' is either whispered, or simply mouthed. Finally, the word 'Stop!' need only be thought. A useful addition to the procedure is the pairing of an unpleasant event with the word 'Stop!'. For example, an elastic band can be pulled, and released against the wrist.

You could go through this sequence of tasks with a member of your family. Alternatively, you could start half way through the conventional procedure, either saying 'Stop!' aloud, or thinking the word 'Stop!' while you release the elastic band against your wrist. Clearly, involving a member of your family might be embarrassing, and you may prefer the latter suggestion.

Although this technique is referred to quite frequently in books on clinical practice, not everyone benefits from its use. As suggested in Chapter 3, there is some evidence to suggest that dismissing or suppressing thoughts can result in their more frequent return at a later stage. For this reason, you should be very careful with this technique. Only use it if you find that stopping thoughts does not result in a distressing 'rebound effect'. In addition, recent research suggests that thought-stopping is more likely to result in improvements if the procedure is applied to the kind of thoughts which occur in response to an obsessional thought, rather than the obsessional thought itself. In other words, it is better to interrupt thought rituals which are employed to reduce anxiety, than to interrupt the obsessional thought that makes you anxious in the first place. By stopping the thoughts that usually make you feel better, you experience your obsessional thought for longer, and this allows habituation to occur.

Having expressed some caution with regard to the use of thought-stopping with obsessional thoughts, one can nevertheless see possible applications of the technique. You may find that in certain situations, for example at work, concentration on the job in hand is essential. If thought-stopping clears your mind, albeit temporarily, then this mind clearance may last long enough for you to complete your task without distraction. Even if your obsessional thought returns with greater frequency later in the day, full concentration might not, then, be at a premium.

Thought-switching and thought-control

It has already been suggested that obsessional thoughts are difficult to control. For the person suffering from uncontrollable thoughts, the recognition of their wayward nature can be associated with several other worries. For example: 'If I can't control my thoughts, then maybe I won't be able to control my behaviour', or 'If I can't control my thoughts, then maybe I'm going mad'. One way of allaying these fears is to provide correct information – i.e. that there is virtually no relationship between obsessional thoughts, acting out their content, and insanity. A second way of allaying these fears is to acquire greater control over mental events by practising 'thought-control' and 'thought-switching'.

Thought-control is accomplished by dismissing your obsessional thought, then trying to re-obtain it. Dismissal might be achieved by employing the thought-stopping procedure described above, or another form of mental distraction. You then repeat the procedure, until you are more confident that the thought doesn't have a 'life of its own'. Clearly, when you first undertake this kind of exercise, control will be difficult; however, with continued practice, you may find that your unruly thoughts can be controlled more easily than expected. This technique is quite attractive for a number of reasons. In particular, you are not attempting to get rid of the thought entirely, which might be unrealistic. Secondly, even partial success is evidence against the belief that you have no control over your own mental processes.

Another similar technique is thought-switching. Write a list of your most troublesome obsessional thoughts. Then write a list of positive alternative thoughts. Here is an example:

I'm going to push somebody over	I'm going to buy a gift
I'm going to swear in public	I'm going to enjoy my holiday
I'm going to kick a dog	I'm going to cuddle my son

Learn the positive thoughts, so that you can summon them up with ease. Try to form your obsessional thought, then practise switching from the obsessional thought to the positive thought immediately. Again, this technique is to give you confidence with regard to the control of mental events; however, you can also use it to provide temporary relief under circumstances where concentration is necessary, and your obsessional thought is distracting.

Coping with worry

'Morbid preoccupations' often take the form of exaggerated concerns, such as having seriously offended someone. Morbid preoccupations are not regarded by the individual as being 'odd', 'absurd' or 'irrational'. Neither are they resisted, in the same way that obsessions are. When they first occur, the individual does not try to block them because they appear strange or unacceptable; indeed they are often quite realistic. Nevertheless, they can be extremely distressing, and in many ways, morbid preoccupations can be compared with extreme worry.

Why worry?

Some commentators have suggested that worry acts like an alarm system, drawing our attention to things going wrong. Although some people say that they worry over nothing, this is probably untrue. What they really mean is that they worry excessively over things which other people might call trivial. Most worry occurs in response to a problem. Therefore, if you are worrying about something, your internal alarm system is telling you that some kind of action is advisable. If you fail to deal with the problem, the alarm will continue to sound until you do.

Coping techniques

If your problem is soluble, then you need to address it as soon as possible. If your problem is insoluble, then you must make efforts to come to terms with it. Psychologists call the first approach 'problem-focused coping', and the second, 'emotion-focused coping'. We will consider each in turn.

Problem-focused and emotion-focused coping

'Problem solving', which is a problem-focused coping strategy, can be undertaken in a systematic way. First, define your problem. Try to specify exactly what it is that you are worrying about. Secondly, try to think up as many alternative solutions to the problem as possible. Don't be critical, just write down as many solutions as come into your head. The reason for this is to give you choice, and to counter any tendency you might have to say: 'Yes, but . . .'; if you say: 'Yes, but . . .' too soon, you will never get the chance to evaluate all your ideas. Thirdly, weigh up the costs and benefits associated with each solution. When you are sure which one is best, try to implement it as soon as possible. Remember, the longer you wait, the more time you'll have to worry in. Finally, evaluate your strategy. Was it successful? If it was, you shouldn't be worrying so much. If it wasn't, then go back to stage two, and select another solution.

'Emotion-focused coping' is about changing your emotional response to a problem where there are no real practical solutions. Insoluble problems are things like past events, death, old age, or an unavoidable surgical operation. Emotion-focused coping is about *coming to terms* with things, rather than finding a solution. It would be wrong to suggest that changing one's emotional response to upsetting circumstances is easy, and a meaningful account of how this might be achieved is really beyond the scope of this book; however, talking things over in a safe environment, and the support of others are usually regarded as being of central importance.

Decatastrophizing

When people worry, they are usually concerned about something bad happening in the immediate future. In the absence of problem-solving, worry can make things seem worse than they really are. It resembles a chain of predictions, where each one is more pessimistic than the last. The persistent prediction of bad outcomes is sometimes called 'catastrophizing'. 'Decatastrophizing' involves breaking out of this chain at the earliest possible opportunity.

Reason generation Worriers are very good at giving reasons for the likely occurrence of unpleasant events; however, they are not so good when it comes to thinking up reasons for the non-occurrence of unpleasant events. In other words, worriers are biased towards the negative. Reasons 'for' catastrophic outcomes seem readily available, but reasons 'against' catastrophic outcomes seem hard to find. One way of breaking out of this pessimistic way of thinking is to practise thinking up reasons why unpleasant outcomes might not happen. For example, if you worry about losing your job, instead of automatically going over the reasons why this might happen, make a list of reasons why it might not happen, such as:

- I am liked by my colleagues; someone would stick up for me;
- It might be considered as unfair dismissal;
- Why should the boss pick on me in particular?

- Although I haven't done well recently, I'm not the worst;
- It would be inconvenient for the company: advertising and training costs would have to be met;
- I did very well last year; that would be taken into account before dismissal.

If you find that you are worrying about the future, challenge every negative prediction by thinking up a reason for why the predicted event might not happen. If you become sufficiently well practised at thinking up both types of reason, 'for' and 'against', then you will have a more balanced view. The idea here is not to convince yourself that bad things are not going to happen (after all, they just might), but rather, to cultivate a *realistic* view of future possibilities. By thinking up reasons against the likelihood of unpleasant events occurring, you might eventually correct your negative bias.

Being realistic If worry makes things seem worse than they actually are, you could try 'tuning in' to the real state of affairs by getting into the habit of asking yourself certain questions like:

- What is the worst thing that can actually happen?
- Would it really be that bad?
- How many times have I thought the worst before?
- How many times have I been wrong?

When we worry we tend to paint a very bleak picture of the future, which we then accept without question. This acceptance can become habitual. If we stop ourselves and question the validity of our predictions, it soon becomes apparent that our concerns are over-exaggerated. For example, many people worry themselves sick over debts; however, in the final reckoning this usually means a minor 'belt tightening' operation and negotiated repayments over a period of several months. At the time, being in debt can seem like a major disaster, but is it really? Will it be relevant in a year's time? In most cases, current worries will be totally forgotten. In summary, try to keep a balanced view of future possibilities, and try to discriminate between actual, and unrealistic possibilities. By using the above techniques, it may be possible to decatastrophize, and reduce preoccupations.

Relaxation

You have probably noticed that when you are upset, or tense, worrying thoughts are more troublesome. They are more difficult to dismiss, and even more difficult to control. It is possible that being tense makes us more 'inward looking'. As a result of this internal focus, we become more aware of our thoughts. If you are feeling tense, then it is likely those thoughts will be unpleasant ones. One way of correcting this internal focus is to reduce the tension. This might be achieved by relaxation exercises (see p. 40). However, informal relaxation might be just as effective. For example, you might prefer to take a warm bath, or prefer listening to relaxing music.

Scheduling 'worry-time'

Another way of coping with worry is to establish a worry period at a particular time each day. Postpone worrying until your worry-time, where you try to solve associated problems. The following instructions might be of some use:

● Learn to identify your worries and preoccupations. Make sure you know the difference between unpleasant thoughts, unnecessary thoughts, and those thoughts which are related to the present moment.
● Establish a half-hour worry period, which is to take place at the same time, and in the same place, every day.
● If you are preoccupied with problems which can actually be dealt with, use your worry period as a time in which you can solve problems. Try to reach a solution at the end of each session, and implement your coping strategy as soon as possible.
● When you find yourself worrying in times outside of your specified half-hour, make a note of your concern, and deal with it at the specified time. When your worries are distracting, try using thought-switching, or just concentrate on present-moment experience.

Summary

1. Exposure to obsessional thoughts can be accomplished by the use of habituation training procedures. The most effective of these involves the employment of a loop tape.

2. Obsessional thoughts often undermine the individual's confidence, with regard to the self-control of mental events. This confidence may be partially repaired by the practice of various thought management procedures. These include thought-stopping, thought-switching, and thought-control.
3. Morbid preoccupations can be compared to extreme worry, and may be responsive to worry management procedures.
4. These include systematic problem solving, decatastrophizing, relaxation, and the postponement of worry to a prearranged worry-period.

10

Managing Obsessional Personality Traits

Many people take issue with the whole notion of personality disorder. We are all different from each other, and the presence of certain characteristics does not automatically suggest a psychiatric illness. However, there is some evidence to suggest that a group of obsessional personality characteristics do 'hang together' in a relatively consistent way, and further, that these can overlap with obsessive–compulsive disorder. If these characteristics interfere with everyday life, or prove to be the source of conflict with other people, then there is, perhaps, an argument for change. In it's pure form obsessive–compulsive personality disorder is asymptomatic, i.e. there are no obsessional complaints (like checking and washing); however, many people with obsessive–compulsive disorder present their GP with personality traits which are consistent with those described under the obsessive–compulsive personality disorder heading.

Personality disorders, in general, can be understood in terms of deeply entrenched habits and beliefs. Because these habits and beliefs are so deeply entrenched, change can be extremely difficult. Efforts to change are often characterized by a pattern of good intentions, followed by back-sliding. Such a pattern can be very frustrating, especially if the individual is seeking a permanent treatment.

Given this, it is probably best to concentrate on the *management* of obsessive–compulsive personality disorder symptoms, rather than on their treatment. Nobody expects to rid themselves of colds completely; you will always get another one. However, you may find that, over time, eating properly and reducing stress makes you less vulnerable to infection. In other words, you adopt a way of coping, rather than attempting cure. Similarly, it is probably unrealistic to expect a 'treatment' for deeply entrenched habits and beliefs; however, over time, you might practise managing your personality difficulties, to the extent that they are less of a problem. Some general comments are provided here, as a rough guide to coping with a few of the more common obsessional traits. They should be considered as suggestions, and nothing more. If you decide to take up some of these suggestions, discussing your progress with a friend might be useful. Another person's point of view can be very helpful, especially if you have fairly rigid ideas about what is right and wrong.

Perfectionism

The most significant obsessional trait is perhaps extreme perfectionism. This involves the setting of high standards, which are often impossible to meet. The individual feels compelled to do things 'absolutely right'. Failure to do so results in feelings of discomfort or dissatisfaction. A common consequence of perfectionism is that tasks are never completed; instead, they are abandoned half-way through, because of disappointment. Alternatively, a task may be repeated over and over again, in a relentless effort to meet impossible standards. One possible way of dealing with this problem is gradually to increase your tolerance for less-than-perfect accomplishments. This can be achieved by adapting the graded hierarchy approach described earlier (see Chapter 4).

When undertaking a particular task, have a clear idea of what would constitute a 'perfect' performance; make a list of all the attributes which would be necessary for a performance to be 'perfect'. Be as concrete as you can. Accomplish each aspect of the task to your usual high standard, with the exception of one. When you have to undertake another task, list all the features of a perfect performance, and accomplish each, with the exception of two. With the next task, leave three imperfect, and so on.

You are not being asked to do things badly; you are being asked to relax your stringent criteria. Try to estimate what would be considered acceptable by the average person. Observing other people is a simple way of doing this. Relax your criteria to the extent that your performance is comparable to the average person, or a little above that, if you are too uncomfortable with the idea of being average. Although, at the end of the day, you won't be able to say: 'This is perfect', at least you will have completed the job in hand. It is better to finish something to a *relatively* high standard, than not finish something at all. Many people who have perfectionist tendencies, are convinced that a less-than-perfect performance will be spotted immediately; however, this is usually not the case. For example, you might re-write a letter only once, instead of four times, or spend ten minutes cleaning the sink instead of 15. See if anybody notices the difference; the absence of criticism could be very persuasive.

Preoccupation with detail

Preoccupation with detail is another obsessional trait which might be managed in a fairly straightforward way. Before undertaking any task, first try to determine what the main point of the task is. If you're about to do the washing up, for example, remind yourself that the main purpose of the exercise is to wash the plates, dry them, and then put them away; it is not to clean the draining board, polish the knives and forks, and then order them in your drawers. Before undertaking anything at all, ask yourself, what's the main point, and only do things which relate to it directly.

Indecisiveness

Indecisiveness can be modified by employing a self-pacing procedure. You will remember that this was discussed in Chapter 8. Make a list of everyday decisions, then rate them for importance. Take the least important decision and try to make it as quickly as you can. Set yourself a reasonable time limit beforehand. You will undoubtedly feel dissatisfied with your decision and feel that you have been careless or hasty. Never mind, just tolerate the discomfort. You will probably find that the outcome is not that different had you sat down and worried over the problem for hours. You can start practising this technique under circumstances where your decision is completely unrelated to a bad outcome. For example, you could go into a book shop and decide to buy a book within 10 minutes. You may not buy the book that will give you most enjoyment, but does that really matter? Presumably, your choice will be enjoyable all the same. A quick decision may not be the *best* decision, but it can still be a *good* one; further, a quick decision is much better than no decision at all – or hours of procrastination when the outcome will be roughly the same anyway. Research has shown that some decisions, made after hours of deliberation, are no better than those made in a relatively short space of time.

Difficulty seeing the other person's point of view and expressing emotion

Another characteristic associated with obsessive–compulsive personality disorder is not being able to see the other person's point of view. When you are involved in some conflict, try taking a break, and then imagining you are the other person. Try to imagine what it is that s/he is feeling, and what it is that s/he wants. Try to argue from her/his point of view, taking into consideration her/his needs. The point here is to increase your power to identify with others. The ability to identify with others, and flexibility, are extremely important attributes where intimate relationships are concerned. This brings us to another problem associated with obsessive–compulsive personality disorder, which is a difficulty expressing emotion.

If you have difficulties with emotional expression, then set yourself modest goals. You can start off with simple things, like accepting compliments. You might say something like: 'Thank you, I appreciate that', or 'It's kind of you to say that'. Similarly, giving compliments to others is easily accomplished and warmly appreciated. In addition, consider how your whole body can sometimes express emotion. For example, the way you stand, the way you sit, the look on your face, and whether or not touch is one of your gestures. Some people feel things very deeply, but it would be impossible to detect that depth of feeling by observation alone. It is as though they are trapped in an exterior which is unresponsive to their changing feelings. Become aware of any discrepancies between what you feel, what you do, and what you say. Try to increase the correspondence gradually, by increasing your general self-awareness.

Understanding others, and the expression of emotion are intimately linked. It is likely that any change in one will effect the other. The more you understand others, the more confident you will be with regard to the expression of feelings. Similarly, the more expressive you are, the more responsive people will be, enabling you to see their point of view.

Devotion to work

Finally, many people who are alleged to have obsessive–compulsive personality disorder are extremely devoted to their work. An excessive devotion to work can leave family, and friends, feeling unloved and uncared for. For those without families and friends, an excessive devotion to work may be instrumental in maintaining their social isolation. If you feel that you are getting too involved in your work, then try to set reasonable goals for the future. For example: 'I will try to reduce my working hours by a quarter by this time next year'. Then, work out ways of achieving this goal in small stages. If you reduce your working hours, then use your extra time constructively: Hobbies, relaxation, travel, family, and developing relationships, are obvious considerations. A general intention to work less is unlikely to be effective. Set yourself concrete goals which are to be achieved in set times.

Summary

1. The cluster of characteristics that are listed under the heading of obsessive–compulsive personality disorder do not necessarily represent a psychiatric problem; however, they may be problematic.
2. Obsessional personality traits are best treated within therapy. Nevertheless, some are associated with behaviours that might be modified using a behavioural approach. Increasing tolerance for discomfort in stages is of central importance.
3. Simple behavioural techniques might be supplemented by exercises employed to increase self-awareness, and awareness of others.
4. Perfectionism, preoccupation with detail, indecisiveness, inability to identify with others, difficulty expressing emotion, and excessive devotion to work, are all obsessive–compulsive personality disorder characteristics which might be profitably modified using simple and straightforward strategies.

11

Coping with Concurrent Depression

Please note, the suggestions in this chapter are for people whose principal problem is obsessive–compulsive disorder. You can use some of these suggestions while undertaking your exposure therapy and response-prevention programme. This chapter should not be viewed as a treatment programme for depression, where depression is the principal problem.

Depression and obsessive–compulsive disorder

Many people with obsessive–compulsive disorder also complain of depression. Three broad categories of sufferers have been identified: 'Keepers', are people who show obsessional symptoms before the onset of a depressive illness, and continue to show obsessional symptoms throughout the course of their depressive illness. 'Losers', are those whose obsessional symptoms gradually disappear after the onset of a depressive illness. Finally, 'Gainers', are those individuals who experience obsessional thoughts and behaviours for the first time during a depressive illness.

The presence of a concurrent depression can make the obsessive–compulsive disorder more difficult to treat. First, because of the effect of mood on thinking: it is possible that when an individual is depressed, unhelpful thoughts become more accessible, and these tend to 'strengthen' the obsessional thoughts; second, it might be that when depressed, individuals feel less motivated to do their homework assignments, and fail to engage in their exposure and response prevention programmes. Either way, the depression usually needs some attention.

In this chapter we will be considering some strategies to help you with mild concurrent depression. If you are very depressed, then it is probably best if you get some professional help. If, for example, you are waking early in the morning, losing your appetite, unable to concentrate, and cannot gain any pleasure from life, then speak to your GP. He or she will be able to refer you on to an appropriate specialist. Some types of depression are responsive to medication and can be relieved fairly swiftly. More tenacious forms of depression can be helped by a combination of psychological therapy and medication. If you have thoughts about taking your own life, then please seek help immediately.

Depression and behaviour

When most people are feeling down, they try to pull themselves out of it by doing pleasant things, like going to the cinema, going out for a meal, or visiting friends. However, when you feel depressed, engaging in the simplest of activities can seem extremely difficult, and this can lead to further worsening of mood. In this way, depression can be regarded as a vicious circle: the more depressed you are, the less likely you are to engage in any pleasant activities, and the less pleasant activities you undertake, the more depressed you feel. It is necessary, therefore, to break out of this vicious circle as soon as possible.

Activity – any kind of activity – is extremely important. It can take your mind off of depressing thoughts and give you a sense of regaining control over your life. Further, the more activities you undertake, the more likely you are to experience some enjoyment, which will counter your depressed mood. Under normal circumstances, when you feel tired, it's a good idea to rest; however, when you are depressed, the exact opposite is true. The more tired, and lethargic you feel, the better it is for you to get up and do something. Finally, there is some evidence to suggest that being active (especially physically) brings about chemical changes in the brain which help to improve mood.

Activity schedule

Getting started is usually the most difficult part, and planning is essential. It's no good making vague resolutions. It is necessary to have a concrete idea of what you are going to do, and when you are going to do it. Constructing an 'activity schedule' can be very helpful. It will reflect your commitment to change, and can go some way towards reducing the stress associated with making decisions at times when you aren't feeling up to it. If you decide to construct an activity schedule, do so when your mood is a little better than usual. All depressions fluctuate. So, do your planning on a 'good day'. Here are some general points to follow:

Activity schedule

Week 1	Time	Activity	Rating
Mon	10.30–11.00 am	Walk in park	P2 A1
Tues			
Wed	1.30– 3.30 pm	Walk in park	P2 A2
Thur			
Fri			
Sat	7.15–10.30 pm	Go to cinema	P5 A4
Sun			
Week 2			
Mon	10.30–11.00 am	Walk in park	P4 A3
Tues	7.30– 9.00 pm	Visit friend	P6 A7
Wed			
Thur			
Fri	2.00– 3.00 pm	Walk in park	P5 A3
Sat			
Sun	3.00– 6.00 pm	Visit family	— —
Week 3			
Mon	10.30–11.30 am	Go swimming	— —
Tues			
Wed	1.30– 2.30 pm	Eat out	— —
Thur	1.30– 2.30 pm	Walk in park	— —
Fri			
Sat	7.15–10.30 pm	Cinema with friend	— —
Sun			

Select a number of activities that you think you might enjoy. Some people say that when they feel depressed, they can't think of anything to do. If you look at the back of this book (Appendix IV) you will find a long list of activities. This may be helpful if nothing immediately comes to mind. This list contains sedentary activities, like reading, as well as more energetic activities, for example participating in sports. Any activity counts, as the accomplishment of each will require motivation, and engender a sense of achievement. Obviously, you don't have to choose something off this list if you already have your own ideas.

Consider one or two activities that you have enjoyed in the past. Try to select those that you think you will find easy. It's important that you don't choose anything too difficult at the beginning, so as to increase your chances of success. Further, try to select activities that are practical. There's little point, for example, in scheduling a skiing holiday if you can't afford it! Another way of increasing the likelihood of success is to organize activities that you know are difficult to 'back out' of – for example, a game of squash with a friend, or a visit to the theatre: if you have already booked a court, or paid for a ticket, you are more likely to go ahead. When you have completed your activity, give it a rating between 0 and 10 for pleasure (P), and sense of achievement (A). Do your rating immediately after completing your activity. If you leave your rating until later, your depressed mood may influence your recollection of events. You might feel that you didn't have such a good time after all, and dismiss your personal achievement. A record can serve to remind you of how you felt at the time – when activity would have been having it's greatest effect. Secondly, improvement might be slow, and gradual. A record will also allow you to detect small changes. Without a record of these small changes you might think that activity was having no effect, and abandon your efforts. This would be a great shame if you were actually making progress, however slow. An example of a three-week activity schedule is shown below. Pleasure and achievement ratings are shown up to half-way through Week 2.

Persevere

If, at first, you find that you don't enjoy your activities, then try to stick with them all the same. Pleasure, like relaxation (see Chapter 4), doesn't necessarily come without effort. Many things that we enjoy in life have to be practised a little. Playing a musical instrument can be extremely gratifying, yet nobody expects to be able to master the violin or the piano in a day. Similarly, appreciating a beautiful poem, or a great work of art, may take several readings or viewings. Undertake your chosen activities regularly, and you may find that your capacity for enjoyment increases over time. If necessary, perform your activities 'mechanically' at first.

Answer back

Another way of increasing your chances of success is to prepare answers to likely discouraging thoughts. This is more or less the same as the self-instruction technique described earlier (see

99

Chapter 5). For example, just before going out you may think to yourself 'I really don't want to do this'. In which case, have a prepared answer already written down on a flash-card. Something like 'Yes, I know that I don't feel like doing this now, but so what? Whether I want to do this, or not, just isn't important. The important thing is that it is in my interests to go. If I do go out, I just might have a good time. If I stay at home, I'll almost certainly do nothing.' Unhelpful thoughts can often come disguised as helpful thoughts, for example: 'I'm really not up to this right now. When I feel a bit better, then I'm more likely to succeed.' To this you could prepare an answer like: 'Yes, when you're feeling better you are more likely to succeed, but you're not going to get better unless you do something about your depression now. Although I don't think I'm up to it right now, I can't really say: after all, I haven't tried, so how can I be so sure!'

Finally, don't dismiss your attempts at activating yourself as unimpressive or negligible. You have to start somewhere, so even a small achievement is better than nothing. For someone immobilized by depression, the first step is the most important of all. Don't undervalue it.

Cognitive therapy techniques

We have already mentioned cognitive therapy several times before. In fact, when cognitive therapy was originally developed it was employed exclusively for the treatment of depression. It is only relatively recently that its broader application has been recognized.

Cognitive therapy is usually undertaken with the help of a therapist; however, the basic principles can be applied within a self-help framework. (If you find some of the suggestions in this section useful, it might be worth reading more about cognitive therapy. Further reading is suggested at the end of this book.)

Negative automatic thoughts

The cognitive model of depression assumes that a particular thinking style is the primary cause of depression. In therapy, the individual is taught to recognize negative automatic thoughts (or NATs for short). They are termed 'negative', because thought content often reflects a poor self-image and a rather pessimistic view of the future. They are termed 'automatic', because such thoughts are not arrived at by reasoning or judgement. As a consequence, they are usually *inaccurate*, but are nevertheless *treated as facts*. Acceptance of, or belief in, these thoughts, is directly related to the experience of depression. The main characteristics of NATs are listed below.

Negative automatic thoughts:

- 'Just happen', as though by reflex. They usually require no effort, which has led to them being described as 'thoughtless thoughts'.
- They are difficult to control. Once you become aware of them, they are not easily dismissed.
- They do not arise from reasoning about the situation(s) in which they occur. Nor do they follow any logical sequence, as might be expected if they were part of a process like problem-solving, i.e. they don't seem to lead anywhere if you reflect on them.
- They are usually accompanied by an unpleasant emotion, in the present case, depression.
- They sometimes occur in short-hand form. For example, instead of thinking: 'It was really stupid of you to say that. David won't talk to you again, now that you've offended him', you might get something like 'Stupid . . . he's offended . . . he'll reject me'.
- They usually seem very plausible at the time, and are treated as though they are facts.
- They can occur in spite of evidence to the contrary.

As we have already said, NATs are usually incorrect. If you were to look at a long list of NATs volunteered by different people you would see that many of them could be grouped together under headings which reflect particular kinds of thinking mistake. For example, there might be a whole group of NATs to do with 'taking the blame for things', while another group might have a lot to do with 'getting things out of proportion'. Although the NATs might be different in themselves, those listed under each heading would reflect the same kind of mistake. These mistakes are called 'thinking errors', and most people have one or two which they commit fairly frequently. There are a number of thinking errors which are easily identified. The less technical ones are listed below. This list is by no means comprehensive, and is simply given as a rough guide, so that you might get a 'flavour' of the concept.

All-or-nothing thinking or black-and-white thinking, is being

101

unable to see the middle ground. Events tend to be interpreted at two extremes, either wonderful or awful. If something isn't perfect then it's a complete and utter failure.

Overgeneralization is taking one negative event, and making far too much of it. For example, if you have a misunderstanding with someone you like, you might overgeneralize in the following way: 'She doesn't really care about me. I doubt whether she ever has. Thinking about it, I don't think anybody has ever cared for me, and I'm beginning to doubt whether anybody ever will.'

Magnification and minimization are two thinking errors which tend to go together. The first is magnifying the importance of unpleasant events, while the second is minimizing the importance of pleasant events. So, you might find yourself dwelling on some small oversight at work, while dismissing the year's achievements.

Personalization is seeing yourself as the main cause of some external misfortune or problem over which you have no real control. This involves seeing connections that really don't exist, and in the end saying 'It's my fault', when there is no justification for such a conclusion.

Objectives

Cognitive therapy involves identifying your most common NATs, and recognizing the kind of thinking errors you are making. If you become aware that you are always magnifying the significance of unpleasant events, or always blaming yourself unnecessarily, then you will be more able to 'catch yourself' making the error in future, and evaluate situations more objectively. That being said, the main task of cognitive therapy involves the identification of NATs. This isn't as easy as it might seem at first. As suggested above, NATs can sometimes occur in a shortened form, and their entrance into, and exit from the mind, may be very swift. Consequently individuals often experience a depressive episode which is apparently inexplicable.

Negative automatic thoughts diary

A much easier way of identifying your NATs is to keep a *Negative automatic thoughts diary*. Make a note of when you are feeling depressed, and try to write down what's going through your mind at the time. This doesn't have to be extensive, and a few summary

COPING WITH CONCURRENT DEPRESSION

statements will do. After a week or two you might be able to detect certain patterns. For example, a particular thought might be more frequent than others, or collectively, your thoughts might reflect a single thinking error. The most useful lesson you will learn, however, is that your mood, and your thoughts, are intimately related. An example of a basic NATs diary is shown below.

Negative automatic thoughts diary

Date	Emotion(s)	Situation	Automatic thoughts
12/9	Sadness	At home, alone	No one loves me
			I have no friends
			This is terrible
13/9	Anxiety	Made mistake at work	I'll get fired
			I look stupid
			I'm incompetent
	Despair	At home, thinking about mistake	I don't deserve to be employed
			I'm worthless
			I'm a fraud

That thoughts and feelings are closely related is really nothing more than common-sense. If you sit and think about a holiday you really enjoyed, or an evening out with friends, it is very likely that your spirits will rise a little. On the other hand, if you sit down and start thinking about a funeral you once attended, or a bad argument you once had, you are going to feel quite bad. What you think will directly influence what you feel.

Challenging your negative automatic thoughts

After monitoring your NATs, you will be able to recognize them when they occur. The next stage of cognitive therapy involves challenging unhelpful thoughts. Challenging involves questioning the validity of your NATs, instead of accepting them as facts. There are a number of challenging questions which have proved to be particularly useful. Here are a few of the more important ones:

• What is the evidence for my thought? Rather than just accepting your thought as a fact, treat it like a speculative statement that can't be accepted without sufficient proof. Evaluate the evidence for it, and against it. If your thought is a NAT, then by definition, you will find that evidence in favour of the thought is rather flimsy.

- Am I being one sided? Are there any alternative interpretations?

  Get into the habit of asking yourself these questions when you interpret a particular event in a negative way. For example, if somebody you know quite well doesn't smile at you, this event might provoke an automatic thought like 'He doesn't like me any more'. Don't accept this interpretation of the event, challenge it! Ask yourself: 'How would another person see this? What is an alternative explanation?' A more accurate explanation might be: 'Although he didn't smile at me, I've got no reason to believe that he was offended. He probably had other things on his mind.'

- What is the effect of thinking the way I do? Appreciate the effect that your thinking has on your mood. Recognize that jumping to conclusions, condemning yourself, and focusing on the negative can only make you feel worse.

Once you have started to question the validity of your thoughts, try replacing them with rational, and unbiased responses. For example, if you automatically think that you are to blame for something, then challenge this, and try to replace it with a more rational response. Something like: 'Yes, things went wrong today. Although I might be partly to blame, I am not to blame entirely.' If you think that you are worthless, try to replace it with something like: 'I only feel worthless because of my depression. I know that some of my friends value my company.' The important thing about your replacement thoughts is that they are accurate and unbiased.

The idea is not simply to 'think positive'. Although a positive outlook is generally recommended, thinking positive irrespective of circumstances is not. If things are genuinely bad, then thinking positive will not be helpful. It will be necessary to recognize the problem, and then undertake some kind of systematic problem-solving. Cognitive therapy seeks to correct negative bias, where it exists. The purpose of cognitive therapy is to encourage an accurate appraisal of circumstances, not to replace a negative bias with a positive one instead.

Once you get the hang of challenging your NATs, and then replacing them with accurate, more rational thoughts, try to keep a full diary. A copy is included in Appendix III for your use. In this diary, rate the degree to which you believe your thoughts before, and after, challenging them. With practice, you will begin to detect changes in degree of belief. As your NATs seem less and less plausible, you will gradually experience an improvement in mood.

Summary

1. Many people with obsessive–compulsive disorder also complain of depression.
2. Mild depression can be addressed in a self-help framework.
3. Increased activity is usually accompanied by a lift in mood. Activity levels can be increased by planning. This is usually accomplished by the use of activity schedules.
4. Depressive thinking can be modified by the use of cognitive therapy techniques. These involve monitoring negative automatic thoughts, and challenging them through a discipline of self-questioning. Eventually, negative biases are corrected, and negative thinking is superseded by more accurate thinking.
5. Self-help techniques are only recommended in mild cases of depression. Severe depression should be treated with the assistance of a health professional.

12

Maintaining Gains, Coping with Setbacks and Alternatives to Self-help

Overcoming problems is rarely straightforward; progress does not always continue at a steady rate. Irregular progress can be very frustrating, too, and you may begin to feel that you are getting nowhere. At times like these, it is important to remind yourself of your overall improvement. Further, that some progress, however modest, is better than no progress at all. If you reach an impasse, try to increase your number of exposure and response-prevention sessions. You may need an intensive day or two to break through the barrier.

If you are successful, and find that your obsessive–compulsive disorder symptoms eventually disappear, then it will be necessary to take precautions to protect your treatment gains. Efforts directed towards prevention of relapse are an essential part of treatment. Although you might feel 'cured', it is wiser to consider yourself in remission. Try not to think of obsessive–compulsive disorder as an illness to be cured, but rather, a problem that can be managed. This has two advantages: first, you need not consider yourself as a 'sick' person, in the same way that someone with arthritis might be considered sick; and second, you will be more likely to protect any progress that you have made through the practice of self-help strategies.

From now on, you are your own therapist, using a repertoire of acquired skills. These can be used not only to manage your obsessive–compulsive disorder, but also to prevent relapse, i.e. a future worsening of symptoms. To ensure that a relapse doesn't occur, it is important not only to practise your newly acquired skills, but also to keep general stress levels down.

Maintaining gains

If you are able to treat your own obsessive–compulsive disorder symptoms, then don't be too complacent about your progress. Occasionally undertake one of your more difficult exposure and response-prevention exercises, just to keep your hand in. Sometimes, symptoms can threaten to re-emerge when unavoidable stress occurs. Therefore, it is extremely useful to be prepared. You may need to repeat certain exercises at regular intervals. This is not an admission of failure. As suggested above, if you regard obsessive–compulsive disorder as a problem, rather than an illness, then there is no need to effect a final cure. Obsessive–compulsive disorder can be managed, in the same way that you would manage a business or your home. The management of obsessive–compulsive disorder becomes a part of your everyday life.

Coping with setbacks

If you think in terms of success and failure, you are more likely to give up attempts at managing your obsessive–compulsive disorder. You are only allowing yourself to be one of two things – 'a success' or 'a failure', and there is no middle ground. Try to erase the word 'failure' from your vocabulary, and replace it with the word 'setback'.

Dealing with stress

Stress, can often account for the re-emergence of symptoms, even after treatment gains have been sustained for a considerable length of time. Stressors can be of two kinds. Major life events (for example, bereavement, the loss of a job, or an accident), and daily hassles (for example, traffic jams, financial problems, or domestic arguments). Both can increase your chances of relapse.

Major life events are difficult to control. We can all expect a few major upheavals during the course of a lifetime. Although nothing can be done specifically to protect yourself from major life events, you can try to cultivate sufficient social contacts to provide support when the need occurs. Family, friends and even casual acquaintances can be the source of enormous comfort when the need to talk arises.

Daily hassles might be reduced by adopting a systematic problem-solving approach (see Chapter 9). You will remember that this involves defining your problems, thinking up solutions, and implementing them as soon as you can. Remember, if you are worried about something, treat your worry as helpful, rather than harmful. Treat your worry as an alarm system that is telling you to engage in active problem-solving. Don't let your worry lead to more worry. Whenever you find yourself worrying, stop! Define the problem, and work towards a solution. Don't let problems build up until they overwhelm you.

Although excessive stress is to be avoided, there is nothing wrong with a little stress. To expect a totally stress-free life is unrealistic. The challenge of a stressful situation, and the satisfaction gained from coping with it, can be very rewarding. Increased self-confidence, and feelings of well being, often accompany such achievements.

Alternatives to self-help

If you have completed the exercises described in this book, and there isn't much improvement, what should you do? First of all, don't give up! There are a number of alternatives available to you, and we will consider each of these in turn.

Seeing a cognitive–behaviour therapist

This book has been primarily about self-help; however, if self-help hasn't been as effective as you had hoped, then you can still see a therapist. The kind of treatment described in this book is called cognitive–behaviour therapy, and it is available on the NHS. You could get a referral from your GP to see a psychiatrist, who would most probably arrange for you to see a clinical psychologist. As suggested in Chapter one, most people with obsessive–compulsive disorder are reluctant to present themselves to their GP because they are embarrassed about their symptoms; however, there really is no need to be embarrassed. Most clinicians have experience of treating obsessive–compulsive disorder, and, there may be over a million people in the UK with this problem, so you are neither odd nor unusual!

Going to see a therapist can be very helpful, especially if you have trouble motivating yourself. Therapists can act like coaches, urging you to do better, while providing appropriate support. Most patients develop a good rapport with their therapists, and actually look forward to their weekly or fortnightly visits. Each session will last for about an hour, and you might be offered anything from 5 to 20 sessions. Although it is impossible to say exactly how successful cognitive–behavioural therapy is, studies show that some improvement can be expected in approximately 60 to 80 per cent of cases.

Seeing other therapists

In addition to cognitive–behavioural therapy, there are a number of other therapeutic approaches which you might find useful, for example, family therapy, or formal psychotherapy. However, as a general rule, it might be more appropriate to try cognitive-behaviour therapy first. This approach does have the best record with regard to the treatment of obsessive–compulsive disorder, as well as related anxiety problems.

Medication

If so called 'psychological therapies' are ineffective, then your GP might suggest medication. Medication can be used on its own, or in conjunction with a psychological approach like cognitive–be-havioural therapy. In many ways, the two approaches are comple-mentary. Recently, there has been a great deal of interest in a group of anti-depressant drugs which appear to help obsessive–compul-sive disorder as well. These are collectively known as the 'serotonin-re-uptake inhibitors'. Serotonin is one of the chemicals in the brain that may be involved in obsessive–compulsive disorder. When these drugs work, upsetting thoughts and compulsive urges, seem to gradually become less intense. The three main drugs in this group are clomipramine (trade name Anafranil), fluoxetine (Prozac), and fluvoxamine (Faverin). There are a number of studies which show that these drugs (especially clomipramine), are more effective than straightforward antidepressants, however, they are associated with some side effects. These include dry mouth, feeling sleepy, blurred vision, constipation, nausea, difficulty urinating, racing heart, sweating, tremor, rashes, temporary impotence, and weight change. Most people, understandably, get quite frightened at the idea of side effects which, although common, need not necessarily be severe. Unfortunately, response cannot be predicted beforehand. Further, each drug has to be taken for about three to twelve weeks before its effectiveness can be evaluated.

Drugs, like psychological approaches, don't necessarily work for everyone. Nevertheless, if your symptoms are causing you distress, and psychological approaches aren't working for you, medication may be worth a try. Recently, the serotonin-re-uptake inhibitors have been used in combination with other drugs which sometimes have the effect of increasing their effectiveness. These include lithium, and the amino acid L-tryptophan. If you experience a partial improvement to clomipramine or one of its relatives, then this might be helped by supplementary medication; however, needless to say, mixing drugs can be associated with further side-effects.

Diet and alternative medicine

Manipulation of your internal chemical environment need not only be achieved through taking medication. You can also do it by changing eating habits. Some time ago, an academic paper was published reporting the treatment of a chronic ruminator by adding a high-protein breakfast to his daily diet. Lasting therapeutic gains were achieved, where all other interventions had proved ineffective. There is a considerable literature on the role of diet in psychological disturbance. Perhaps the most famous is that which makes a connection between certain foods, certain food additives, and the occurrence of hyperactivity in children. If your obsessive–compulsive disorder proves unresponsive to all of the interventions described in this book, then dietary change might be advisable. Alternative practitioners, like clinical ecologists, might be the best people to consult if you find the idea attractive.

Although there are few scientific investigations into the efficacy of alternative approaches, it would be premature to dismiss them out of hand. Many of the drugs used in medical practice are derived from plants and flowers, and it may be the case that some of the so-called natural remedies are just as effective. You may want to explore some of these yourself. In Bach flower therapy, for example, White Chestnut is alleged to be helpful with unwanted thoughts.

In conclusion, this book has concentrated on a particular psychological approach. Although this approach has an extremely good record with regard to the treatment of obsessive–compulsive disorder, you should recognize that a wide range of treatments are available.

Summary

1. The successful preservation of treatment gains is best achieved by adopting a number of relapse-prevention strategies.
2. It is extremely important to recognize the role of stress in relapse. Stress management, or lifestyle change, may be necessary to preserve treatment gains.

3. If self-help is not effective, a number of options remain. These include consulting a cognitive–behaviour therapist, a psychotherapist, or a family therapist.
4. Medication can be helpful on its own, or taken in conjunction with a 'psychological treatment'.
5. Diet change, and consulting alternative practitioners can be entertained, if conservative practice is ineffective.

Glossary

Clinical

To do with medicine/illness/therapy.

Clinical psychology

The speciality of psychology dealing with mental illness and distress and its treatment using non-drug methods.

Cognitive

To do with thinking and thought processes.

Cognitive therapy

A form of psychotherapy in which the patient is encouraged to change the way he/she thinks by systematic self-questioning.

Exposure therapy

A form of psychotherapy where the patient is encouraged to tolerate being exposed to feared things or situations. It is usually undertaken in gradual stages.

Habituation

The process by which we become accustomed to repeated events and therefore no longer react to them in the same (strong) way.

Psychiatry

The medical speciality dealing with mental disorder and its diagnosis and treatment.

Psychology

The scientific study of human and animal behaviour.

Psychotherapy

The non-drug alleviation of mental and emotional distress. There are many forms of psychotherapy.

Therapy

Means 'treatment' but is also used loosely to mean psychotherapy.

Further Reading

Other books that might be useful:

On anxiety
Marks, I. (1978). *Learning to Live with Fear: Understanding and Coping with Anxiety*. New York, McGraw Hill.

On worry
Tallis, F. (1990). *How to Stop Worrying*. Sheldon Press, London.

On stress
Fontana, D. (1989). *Managing Stress*. British Psychological Society/ Routledge, Leicester.
Parry, G. (1990). *Coping with Crises*. British Psychological Society/ Routledge, Leicester.

On depression and cognitive therapy
Rowe, D. (1983). *Depression: The Way Out of Your Prison*. Routledge, London.
Burns, D. (1981). *Feeling Good: The New Mood Therapy*. Willam Morrow and Co., New York.

I have avoided the use of extensive footnotes and references. The following books and articles provided important source material:

Chapter 1
Myers, J. K., Weissman, M. M., Tischler, G. L., Holzer, C. E., Leaf, P. J., Orvaschel, H., Anthony, J. C., Boyd, J. H., Burke, J.D., Kramer, M. and Stoltzman, R. (1984). Six-month prevalence of psychiatric disorders in three communities. *Archives of General Psychiatry* **41**, 959–67.
Pollak, J. M. (1979). Obsessive–compulsive personality: A review. *Psychological Bulletin* **86**, 225–41.
Rapoport, J. L. (1989). *The Boy who couldn't Stop Washing*. E. P. Dutton, New York.
Young, J. E. (1987). *Schema-Focused Cognitive Therapy for Personality Disorders*. Department of Psychiatry, Columbia University.

Chapter 2

Insel, T. R., Zahn, T. and Murphy, D. L. (1985). Obsessive–compulsive disorder: An anxiety disorder? In *Anxiety and the Anxiety Disorders*, edited by Tuma, A. H. and Maser, J. D. Erlbaum, Hillside, New Jersey.

Marks, I. (1987). *Fears, Phobias and Rituals*. Oxford University Press, New York.

Rachman, S. and Hodgson, R. (1980). *Obsessions and Compulsions*. Prentice Hall, Englewood Cliffs, New Jersey.

Chapter 3

Rachman, S. and de Silva, P. (1978). Abnormal and normal obsessions. *Behavior, Research and Therapy* **16**, 233–48.

Salkovskis, P. M. (1985). Obsessional–compulsive problems: A cognitive–behavioural analysis. *Behavior, Research and Therapy* **22**, 571–83.

Wegner, D. M. (1989). *White Bears and Other Unwanted thoughts: Suppression, Obsession and the Psychology of Mental Control*. Viking, New York.

Chapter 4

Juninger, J. and Head, S. (1991). Time series analysis of obsessional behaviour and mood during self-imposed delay and response prevention. *Behavior, Research and Therapy* **29**, 521–30.

Meyer, V., Levey, R. and Schnurer, A. (1974). The behavioural treatment of obsessive–compulsive disorder. In *Obsessional States*, edited by Beech, H. R. Methuen, London.

Zohar, J., Insel, T., Berman, K., Foa, E., Hill, J. and Weinberger, D. (1989). Anxiety and cerebral blood flow during behavioral challenge. *Archives of General Psychiatry* **46**, 505–10.

Chapter 7

Hussian, R. A. (1980). Stimulus control in the modification of problematic behavior in the elderly. Paper presented at the annual meeting of the Association for the advancement of behavior therapy, New York.

Sher, K., Frost, R., Kushner, M., Crews, T. and Alexander, J. (1989). Memory deficits in compulsive checkers: Replication and extension in a clinical sample. *Behavior, Research and Therapy* **27**, 65–69.

Sher, K., Frost, R. and Otto, R. (1983). Cognitive deficits in compulsive checkers: an exploratory study. *Behavior, Research and Therapy* **21**, 357–63.

Steketee, G. S., Foa, E. B. and Grayson, J. B. (1982). Recent advances in the behavioural treatment of obssesive-compulsives. *Archives of General Psychiatry* **39**, 1365–71.

Toates, F. (1990). *Obsessional Thoughts and Behaviour*. Thorsons, London.

Chapter 8

Rachman, S. and Hodgson, R. (1980). *Obsessions and Compulsions*. Prentice Hall, Englewood Cliffs, New Jersey.

Chapter 9

Barlow, D. (1988). *Anxiety and its Disorders*. The Guilford Press, London.

Borkovec, T., Wilkinson, L., Folensbee, R. and Lerman, C. (1983). Stimulus control applications to the treatment of worry. *Behavior, Research and Therapy* **21**, 247–51.

MacLeod, A., Williams, M. G. and Bekerian, D. A. (1991). Worry is reasonable: The role of explanations in pessimism about future personal events. *Journal of Abnormal Psychology.* **4**, 478–86.

Rachman, S. (1974). Some similarities and differences between obsessional ruminations and morbid preoccupations. *Canadian Psychiatric Association Journal* **18**, 71–4.

Salkovskis, P. M. (1983). Treatment of an obsessional patient using habituation to audiotaped ruminations. *British Journal of Clinical Psychology* **22**, 311–13.

Salkovskis, P. M. and Westbrook, D. (1989). Behaviour therapy and obsessional ruminations: Can failures be turned into success? *Behavior, Research and Therapy* **27**, 149–60.

Tallis, F. and de Silva, P. (1992). Worry and Obsessionality: A correlational analysis. *Behavior, Research and Therapy* **30**, 103–5.

Chapter 11

Gittleson, N. (1966). The fate of obsessions in depressive psychosis. *British Journal of Psychiatry* **112**, 705–8.

Chapter 12

Rapoport, J. L. (1989). *The Boy who Couldn't Stop Washing*. E. P. Dutton, New York.

FURTHER READING

Rippere, V. Dietary treatment of chronic obsessional ruminations. *British Journal of Clinical Psychology* **22**, 314–16.

Appendix I
Self-Assessment Questionnaire

A systematic examination of your most frequent obesessive–compulsive disorder symptoms

(See Chapter 3)

1. What is your most frequent unwanted thought or image?

_____

_____

_____

_____

_____

2. Are there particular times of the day when you get your most frequent unwanted thought or image?

Tick a box

YES ☐   NO ☐

If YES, then *tick a box below* to show when. You can tick more than one box.

Midnight–3am ☐   3–6am ☐   6–9am ☐   9am–Noon ☐
Noon–3pm ☐   3–6pm ☐   6–9pm ☐   9pm–Midnight ☐

3. Are there particular places where you get your most frequent unwanted thought or image? If so, where?

_____

_____

_____

_____

4. Do you avoid these places?

Please put a circle around the number on this scale which reflects the degree to which you avoid these places. Statements are given as a guide under certain numbers. However, you can use the numbers 'in between' as well.

0	1	2	3	4	5	6	7	8
Not at all		Rarely		Sometimes		Often		Always

5. Is your most frequent unwanted thought or image triggered by particular situations, or people? What are these situations? Who are the people?

_____

_____

_____

_____

_____

_____

6. Do you avoid these situations?

0	1	2	3	4	5	6	7	8
Not at all		Rarely		Sometimes		Often		Always

7. Do you avoid these people?

0	1	2	3	4	5	6	7	8
Not at all		Rarely		Sometimes		Often		Always

8. On average, how often do you get your most frequent unwanted thought and image? *Tick an appropriate box*

About once a month .... ☐
About once a fortnight .... ☐
About once a week .... ☐
Maybe once every 2 or 3 days .... ☐
About once a day .... ☐
About twice a day .... ☐
About three times a day .... ☐
About four times a day .... ☐
About five times a day .... ☐
About five and ten times a day .... ☐
Between ten and fifteen times a day .... ☐
Between fifteen and twenty times a day .... ☐
Between twenty and thirty times a day .... ☐

Between thirty and forty times a day .... □
Between forty and fifty times a day .... □
More than fifty times a day .... □
More or less continuously .... □

9. When you get your most frequent unwanted thought or image, for how long, on average, does it stay in your mind?

Tick an appropriate box

Fleeting? □
Seconds? 0–4 □ 5–14 □ 15–30 □ 31–45 □ 46–60 □
Minutes? 1–2 □ 2–5 □ 5–10 □ 10–15 □ 15–30 □ 30–45 □ 45–60 □
Hours? 1–2 □ 2–4 □ 4–6 □ 6–8 □ 8–10 □ 10–12 □ 12+ □

10. Do you find your most frequent unwanted thought or image unacceptable? (i.e. Do you find it disgusting or shameful)

0	1	2	3	4	5	6	7	8

Not at all   A little   Quite   Very   Completely
unacceptable   unacceptable   unacceptable   unacceptable   unacceptabl

11. Do you find your most frequent unwanted thought or image ridiculous? (i.e. Do you find it bizarre or senseless)

0	1	2	3	4	5	6	7	8

Not at all   A little   Quite   Very   Completely
ridiculous   ridiculous   ridiculous   ridiculous   ridiculous

12. When you get your most frequent unwanted thought or image, do you become anxious, tense, or feel discomfort?

0	1	2	3	4	5	6	7	8

Not at all   Rarely   Sometimes   Often   Always

13. How much anxiety, tension, or discomfort do you experience?

0	1	2	3	4	5	6	7	8

None   Slight   Moderate   Marked   Extreme

14. When you get your most frequent unwanted thought or image,

do you feel as though you have to do something to make things right; even though you know that rationally, what you do doesn't really make much of a difference? If so, What do you do?

_____

_____

_____

_____

15. How long does it take you to complete?

Fleeting? ☐
Seconds? 0–4 ☐ 5–14 ☐ 15–30 ☐ 31–45 ☐ 46–60 ☐
Minutes? 1–2 ☐ 2–5 ☐ 5–10 ☐ 10–15 ☐ 15–30 ☐ 30–45 ☐ 45–60 ☐
Hours? 1–2 ☐ 2–4 ☐ 4–6 ☐ 6–8 ☐ 8–10 ☐ 10–12 ☐ 12+ ☐

16. After doing the above, do you feel better?

0	1	2	3	4	5	6	7	8
Not at all better		A little better		No different		Quite better		Much better

17. If you circled 1 or more above, how long, on average, does this feeling of relief last?

Please tick an appropriate box

Fleeting? ☐
Seconds? 0–4 ☐ 5–14 ☐ 15–30 ☐ 31–45 ☐ 46–60 ☐
Minutes? 1–2 ☐ 2–5 ☐ 5–10 ☐ 10–15 ☐ 15–30 ☐ 30–45 ☐ 45–60 ☐
Hours? 1–2 ☐ 2–4 ☐ 4–6 ☐ 6–8 ☐ 8–10 ☐ 10–12 ☐ 12+ ☐

18. Do you ever ask people for reassurance?

Please circle an appropriate number

0	1	2	3	4	5	6	7	8
Not at all		Rarely		Sometimes		Often		Always

19. If you do seek reassurance, does this make you feel better?

Please circle an appropriate number

APPENDIX I

0	1	2	3	4	5	6	7	8
Not at all		Rarely		Sometimes		Often		Always

20. If you circled 1 or above, how long, on average, does this feeling of relief last?

Please tick an appropriate box

Fleeting? ☐
Seconds? 0–4 ☐ 5–14 ☐ 15–30 ☐ 31–45 ☐ 46–60 ☐
Minutes? 1–2 ☐ 2–5 ☐ 5–10 ☐ 10–15 ☐ 15–30 ☐ 30–45 ☐ 45–60 ☐
Hours? 1–2 ☐ 2–4 ☐ 4–6 ☐ 6–8 ☐ 8–10 ☐ 10–12 ☐ 12+ ☐

21. If you tried to stop yourself from doing your compulsive activity, be it mental or physical, how much anxiety, tension or discomfort would you feel?

0	1	2	3	4	5	6	7	8
None		Slight		Moderate		Marked		Extreme

22. On average, do you think that your most frequent unwanted thought or image causes your work performance to be impaired?

0	1	2	3	4	5	6	7	8
Not at all		Slightly		Definitely		Markedly		Very severely: I can't cope

23. On average, do you think that your most frequent unwanted thought or image causes your home life to be impaired (e.g cleaning, shopping etc.)?

0	1	2	3	4	5	6	7	8
Not at all		Slightly		Definitely		Markedly		Very severely: I can't cope

24. On average, do you think that your most frequent unwanted thought or image causes your social and leisure activities to be impaired?

0	1	2	3	4	5	6	7	8
Not at all		Slightly		Definitely		Markedly		Very severely: I can't cope

Appendix II

Instructions for Relaxation

Stage 1: Deep relaxation

Deep relaxation involves tensing, and then relaxing, various muscle groups. When you tense a particular part of your body, hold the tension for anything between 3 and 6 seconds, then relax. Wait for about 20 to 45 seconds, before tensing the next muscle group.

Make sure that you are comfortable – either lying down or sitting, with your legs uncrossed and your hands by your side. Try to do these exercises in a quiet room, when you will not be disturbed. Before starting the sequence of exercises described below, concentrate on your breathing. Every time you breathe out, think of the word *'relax'*. Enjoy the sensation of your lungs filling with air, before breathing out, and thinking *'relax'*. The exercises are as follows. Work down the page. Try to make each deep relaxation session last for about 25 minutes.

1. Hands: Clench, making fists. Release.
2. Biceps (i.e. upper arms): Try to touch shoulders with wrists. Hold. Return to starting position.
3. Forearms: Stretch arms, with fingers outstretched. Hold. Return to starting position.
4. Shoulders: Lift shoulders, as though shrugging. Hold. Return to starting position.
5. Neck: Move head backwards, push against chair or pillow. Hold. Release.
6. Jaw: Clench teeth together. Hold. Release.
7. Lips: Press lips together. Hold. Release.
8. Tongue and throat: Flip tongue backwards, and press against roof of mouth. Hold. Return to usual position.
9. Eyes: Screw up eyes, pressing eyelids together. Hold. Release.
10. Forehead: Lift eyebrows, as though enquiring. Hold. Release.
11. Chest: Take deep breath in. Hold. Exhale slowly.
12. Stomach: Tighten stomach muscles, pulling stomach in. Hold. Release.
13. Hips: Tighten buttocks. Hold. Release.
14. Legs: Stretch legs. Hold. Return to starting position.

15. Feet: Clench. Hold. Release.

Stage 2: Quick relaxation

This involves relaxing the parts of the body listed above but without tensing them first. Try to make a quick relaxation session last for about 10 or 15 minutes.

1. Hands	9. Eyes
2. Biceps	10. Forehead
3. Forearms	11. Chest
4. Shoulders	12. Stomach
5. Neck	13. Hips
6. Jaw	14. Legs
7. Lips	15. Feet
8. Tongue and throat	

Stage 3: Applied relaxation

This is a relaxation technique that you can use while doing other things. Close your eyes. Take a deep breath in. Hold it for about 5 seconds. Then exhale, thinking '*Relax*'. Try to relax your whole body at once.

When you have mastered deep relaxation, move on to quick relaxation. Try using applied relaxation in a situation which usually makes you anxious. Remember, relaxation is a skill. In stage 3, you are being asked to relax your entire body in a matter of seconds. This cannot be achieved without practice.

Appendix III

Self-Help Charts and Diaries

Compulsive Washing and Cleaning: Self-help Programme
(See Chapter 6)

List the situations that cause you discomfort and usually result in an
urge to wash/clean and rate them using the 8-point anxiety scale.

Situations causing discomfort and usually resulting in an urge to wash/clean	Anxiety rating (0–8)
_____	_____
_____	_____
_____	_____
_____	_____
_____	_____
_____	_____
_____	_____
_____	_____
_____	_____
_____	_____
_____	_____
_____	_____
_____	_____
_____	_____
_____	_____
_____	_____
_____	_____
_____	_____
_____	_____
_____	_____
_____	_____
_____	_____
_____	_____
_____	_____
_____	_____
_____	_____
_____	_____
_____	_____

APPENDIX III

Construct a five-step anxiety ladder, and include your anxiety rating for each item.

Anxiety
rating (0–8)

Step 5 _____ _____
Step 4 _____ _____
Step 3 _____ _____
Step 2 _____ _____
Step 1 _____ _____

Construct an exposure and response-prevention plan. With every exposure increase contact, extend delay time and reduce wash time.
What are your contact, delay and wash times?

Exposures	Contact	Time (min) Delay	Wash
12	___	___	___
11	___	___	___
10	___	___	___
9	___	___	___
8	___	___	___
7	___	___	___
6	___	___	___
5	___	___	___
4	___	___	___
3	___	___	___
2	___	___	___
1	___	___	___

APPENDIX III

Washing/Cleaning Diary

Date: ....   Time: ....

Please specify item
(e.g. sink): ....

Goals: Contact time:.......... Delay:.......... Washing time:..........

Time spent delaying wash (Please tick)

Less than 1 minute ☐   About 1 minute   ☐
About 2 minutes   ☐   About 3 minutes   ☐
About 4 minutes   ☐   About 5 minutes   ☐
5–15 min ☐   15–30 ☐   30–45 ☐   45–1 hr ☐
1 hr–1 hr 30 min ☐   1 hr 30 min–2 hr ☐
2–3 hr ☐   3–4 ☐   4–5 ☐   5+ hr ☐
If more than 5 hr, please specify time ....

Discomfort/anxiety (when resisting)

0	1	2	3	4	5	6	7	8
Absent		Slight		Definite		Marked		Extreme

Time spent washing (Please tick)

Less than 1 minute ☐   About 1 minute   ☐
About 2 minutes   ☐   About 3 minutes   ☐
About 4 minutes   ☐   About 5 minutes   ☐
5–15 min ☐   15–30 ☐   30–45 ☐   45–1 hr ☐
1 hr–1 hr 30 min ☐   1 hr 30 min–2 hr ☐
2–3 hr ☐   3–4 ☐   4–5 ☐   5+ hr ☐
If more than 5 hr, please specify time ....

Discomfort/anxiety (after washing)

0	1	2	3	4	5	6	7	8
Absent		Slight		Definite		Marked		Extreme

Compulsive Checking: Self-Help Programme
(See Chapter 7)

List things that you check excessively, and note the
discomfort/anxiety felt by you (using the eight-point
scale) when not able to check these items.
Things checked excessively: Anxiety
                                                rating

_____ _____
_____ _____
_____ _____
_____ _____
_____ _____
_____ _____
_____ _____
_____ _____
_____ _____
_____ _____
_____ _____
_____ _____
_____ _____
_____ _____
_____ _____
_____ _____
_____ _____
_____ _____
_____ _____
_____ _____
_____ _____
_____ _____
_____ _____
_____ _____
_____ _____
_____ _____
_____ _____

Construct a five-step anxiety ladder, and include your anxiety rating for each item.

Step 5 _____ _____
Step 4 _____ _____
Step 3 _____ _____
Step 2 _____ _____
Step 1 _____ _____

Construct an exposure and response-prevention plan, so that with every exposure you reduce the initial number of checks, increase the delay time and reduce the final number of checks.

Exposures	Initial Minor	Major	Time (min) Delay	Final Minor	Major
12					
11					
10					
9					
8					
7					
6					
5					
4					
3					
2					
1					

Checking Diary 1

Date: ....   Time: ....

Please specify item
(e.g. door): ....

Goals:	Initial *Minor*	Check *Major*	Delay time *Minutes*	Final *Minor*	Check *Major*
Number	_____	_____	_____	_____	_____

Time spent checking initially (Please tick)

Less than 1 minute ☐   About 1 minute ☐
About 2 minutes ☐   About 3 minutes ☐
About 4 minutes ☐   About 5 minutes ☐
5–15 min ☐   15–30 ☐   30–45 ☐   45–1 hr ☐
1 hr–1 hr 30 min ☐   1 hr 30 min–2 hr ☐
2–3 hr ☐   3–4 ☐   4–5 ☐   5+ hr ☐
If more than 5 hr, please specify time ....

Discomfort/anxiety (when resisting)

0	1	2	3	4	5	6	7	8
Absent		Slight		Definite		Marked		Extreme

Time spent checking finally (Please tick)

Less than 1 minute ☐   About 1 minute ☐
About 2 minutes ☐   About 3 minutes ☐
About 4 minutes ☐   About 5 minutes ☐
5–15 min ☐   15–30 ☐   30–45 ☐   45–1 hr ☐
1 hr–1 hr 30 min ☐   1 hr 30 min–2 hr ☐
2–3 hr ☐   3–4 ☐   4–5 ☐   5+ hr ☐
If more than 5 hr, please specify time ....

Discomfort/anxiety (after final check)

0	1	2	3	4	5	6	7	8
Absent		Slight		Definite		Marked		Extreme

Checking Diary 2

Date: .... Time: ....

Please specify item
(e.g. door): ....

Goals:	Initial *Minor*	Check *Major*	Delay time *Minutes*	Final *Minor*	Check *Major*
Number	_____	_____	_____	_____	

Number of actual checks

Initial

	Minor	Major		Minor	Major
One	☐	☐	Ten to 15	☐	☐
Two	☐	☐	15 to 20	☐	☐
Three	☐	☐	20 to 25	☐	☐
Four	☐	☐	30 to 40	☐	☐
Five	☐	☐	40 to 50	☐	☐
Six	☐	☐	50 to 75	☐	☐
Seven	☐	☐	75 to 100	☐	☐
Eight	☐	☐	More than 100	☐	☐
Nine	☐	☐	More than 200	☐	☐
Ten	☐	☐	More than 300	☐	☐

Discomfort/anxiety (when resisting)

0	1	2	3	4	5	6	7	8
Absent		Slight		Definite		Marked		Extreme

Number of actual checks

Final

	Minor	Major		Minor	Major
One	☐	☐	Ten to 15	☐	☐
Two	☐	☐	15 to 20	☐	☐
Three	☐	☐	20 to 25	☐	☐
Four	☐	☐	30 to 40	☐	☐
Five	☐	☐	40 to 50	☐	☐
Six	☐	☐	50 to 75	☐	☐
Seven	☐	☐	75 to 100	☐	☐
Eight	☐	☐	More than 100	☐	☐
Nine	☐	☐	More than 200	☐	☐
Ten	☐	☐	More than 300	☐	☐

Discomfort/anxiety (after final check)

0	1	2	3	4	5	6	7	8
Absent		Slight		Definite		Marked		Extreme

Primary Obsessional Slowness: Treatment Plan
(See Chapter 8)

Item _____

Current time taken _____ minutes

Goal time _____ minutes

Sessions	Time allowed (min)
7	___
6	___
5	___
4	___
3	___
2	___
1	___

APPENDIX III

Negative Automatic Thoughts Diary
(See Chapter 11)

Date: ....
1. How depressed did you feel?

0	1	2	3	4	5	6	7	8
Not at all depressed		Slightly depressed		Definitely depressed		Markedly depressed		Severely depressed

2. What were you doing when you felt depressed?

_____
_____
_____

3. What were your automatic thoughts at the time?

4. Could you rate how much you believed them?

0	1	2	3	4	5	6	7	8
No belief		Slight belief		Definite belief		Strong belief		Total belief

Thoughts   *Ratings*
1) _____   _____
_____
2) _____   _____
_____
3) _____   _____
_____

5. What are your rational responses to your automatic thoughts?
1) _____
_____
_____
2) _____
_____
_____
3) _____
_____
_____

6. How much do you believe them now?

0	1	2	3	4	5	6	7	8
No belief		Slight belief		Definite belief		Strong belief		Total belief

1) _____ 2) _____ 3) _____

7. How depressed do you feel now?

0	1	2	3	4	5	6	7	8
Not at all depressed		Slightly depressed		Definitely depressed		Markedly depressed		Severely depressed

Appendix IV

Pleasant Activities

(see Chapter 11)

Talking about my hobby
Being with my partner
Nature walks
Looking after houseplants
Walking
Collecting things
Playing squash
Sewing
Looking after children
Beach-combing
Going to auctions
Going to car-boot sales
Community service
Water skiing
Scuba diving
Reading comics
Hearing sermons
Travelling
Seeing old friends
Office parties
Get-togethers
Attending a concert
Going to the opera
Going to the ballet
Going to the theatre
Seeing a musical
A trip to the country
Contributing to a religious
    group, or charity
Talking about sport
Attending a rock concert
Planning a holiday
Lying on a beach
Painting
Drawing

Making models
Sculpting
Pottery
Rock climbing
Reading Scripture
Playing golf
Rearranging a room
Redecorating
Going to a sports event
Reading books
Going to see a horse race
Going to see a car or motorbike
    race
Going to a bar
Going to a club
Driving
Boating
Hiring a row boat
Restoring antiques
Camping
Car maintenance
Motorcycle maintenance
Playing cards
Cross-word puzzles
Playing tennis
Carpentry
Writing stories
Writing poems
Watching animals
Taking a plane
Exploring (walking away from
    known routes)
Singing in a choir
Going to a party
Going to church functions

Playing a musical instrument
Skiing
Amateur dramatics
Being with friends
Cookery
Making preserves
Going to a city
Playing pool or billiards
Being with grandchildren
Craftwork
Jewellery making
Putting on make-up
Visiting the sick
Buying a present
Photography
Seeing beautiful scenery
Eating out
Playing in a musical group
Hiking
Writing essays or articles
Fishing
Going to a health club
Going to a sauna
Working out in a gym
Learning something new
Visiting parents
Riding
Badminton
Going to the cinema
Family reunions

Reminiscing
Visiting friends
Keeping a diary
Playing football
Meditation
Yoga
Playing board games
Outdoor work
Relaxing
Reading the newspaper
Reading a magazine
Ping-pong
Swimming
Running
Jogging
Playing frisbee
Listening to music
Knitting
Embroidery
Going to the barber
Going to a beautician
Having house-guests
Sex
Going to the library
Playing rugby
Shopping
Repairing things
Cycling
Writing letters
Talking about politics

Appendix V

OCD Action is a charity (formerly called Obsessive Action) for people with obsessive–compulsive disorder and their families. If you would like to know more about OCD Action, please write to the following address, or visit their website:

OCD Action
Suite 506–507 Davina House
137–149 Goswell Road
London
EC1V 7ET
Helpline: 0845 390 6232 / 020 7253 2664
Tel.: 020 7253 5272
Website: www.ocdaction.org.uk

A similar organization exists in the USA:

International OCD Foundation (formerly the **Obsessive Compulsive Foundation**)
P.O. Box 961029
Boston
MA 02196
USA
Tel.: (001) 617 973 5801
Website: www.ocfoundation.org

Index